医务人员实用英语系列
Practical English for Medical Staff Series

# 院前急救医务人员
# 英语手册

## English Handbook for
## Medical Staff at Pre-hospital Emergency

海南省卫生健康委员会　组织编写

窦　岩　韩丽萍　王　飞　编　著

人民卫生出版社
·北京·

**图书在版编目（CIP）数据**

院前急救医务人员英语手册 / 窦岩，韩丽萍，王飞编著 . -- 北京 ：人民卫生出版社，2024. 8. --（医务人员实用英语系列）. -- ISBN 978-7-117-36716-5

Ⅰ. R459.7-62

中国国家版本馆 CIP 数据核字第 2024RT7785 号

| | | |
|---|---|---|
| 人卫智网 | www.ipmph.com | 医学教育、学术、考试、健康，购书智慧智能综合服务平台 |
| 人卫官网 | www.pmph.com | 人卫官方资讯发布平台 |

院前急救医务人员英语手册

Yuanqian Jijiu Yiwu Renyuan Yingyu Shouce

编　　著：窦　岩　韩丽萍　王　飞
出版发行：人民卫生出版社（中继线 010-59780011）
地　　址：北京市朝阳区潘家园南里 19 号
邮　　编：100021
E - mail：pmph @ pmph.com
购书热线：010-59787592　010-59787584　010-65264830
印　　刷：天津科创新彩印刷有限公司
经　　销：新华书店
开　　本：850×1168　1/32　印张：9
字　　数：202 千字
版　　次：2024 年 8 月第 1 版
印　　次：2024 年 11 月第 1 次印刷
标准书号：ISBN 978-7-117-36716-5
定　　价：39.00 元

打击盗版举报电话：010-59787491　E-mail：WQ @ pmph.com
质量问题联系电话：010-59787234　E-mail：zhiliang @ pmph.com
数字融合服务电话：4001118166　E-mail：zengzhi @ pmph.com

# 前　言

　　随着全球经济不断深入融合,医学领域日益频繁的交流与合作,对医务人员的英语水平和沟通能力提出了更高的要求。具备良好英语应用和沟通能力的院前急救医务人员不仅能更好地与国际同行交流,分享急救经验和技术,而且能够快速、准确地与外籍病人/家属沟通,了解病情,为救治争取宝贵的时间。

　　本书以院前急救过程中经常遇到的各种问诊和救治场景为背景,模拟医生与病人/家属之间对话,总结院前急救医务人员常用英语词汇、短语、表达和对话。全书共有7个章节,涵盖内科常见急症、妇产科常见急症、儿科常见急症、环境及理化因素所致常见损伤、常见急性中毒、感染与传染性常见急症以及常见创伤内容。每个章节都紧密结合院前急救实际需求,针对各种急症设置急救场景,提供实用英语单词、短语、表达和对话示例,帮助医务人员在紧急情况下用英语流畅交流。

　　本书具有以下特点:

　　1. 科学性:编写小组精心挑选语言素材,确保其符合院前急救医务人员和相关学习者的认知特点和实际英语水平。同时,充分考虑到医务人员与外籍病人/家属沟通时可能存在的语言困难,采用容易理解的简单会话作为学习材料,提供相关的词语、句型供学习者借鉴和反复操练。

　　2. 实用性:本书旨在提高院前急救医务人员在工作中运用英语的能力。内容紧密结合常见的医疗场景和急救任务,提供实用的英语表达方式和词汇,方便医务人员在紧急情况下快速、准确地与外籍病人/家属进行沟通。同时,本书还有利于培养医务人员的开放意识、外语文化素养和跨文化交际能力。

3. 针对性:本书主要针对院前急救医务人员这一特定群体,重点突出急救场景下的英语应用,更加注重医务人员在医疗工作中的口语表达,以满足院前急救医务人员在实际抢救工作中的英语沟通需求,可供不同水平的学习者反复操练,提高自身英语水平。

在编写过程中,编写小组严格遵循科学性、实用性和针对性的原则,经过广泛收集资料、深入调研和多次讨论,逐步确定本书的结构和内容。本书由窦岩总统筹,韩丽萍编写第一、二章,王飞编写第三章到第七章。

本书主要服务院前急救医务人员,同时适用于广大临床医护人员、急诊医学专业的学生以及其他希望提高医学英语水平的人士。无论是在国际救援任务中,还是在国内医疗机构中接待外籍病人/家属时,本书都能为您提供有力的语言支持。

在编写过程中,我们得到了许多同行和专家的无私帮助和支持,在此表示衷心的感谢。尽管我们付出最大努力,但书中难免存在疏漏和不足之处,恳请广大读者批评指正。

窦岩　韩丽萍　王飞

2024 年 3 月

# Contents

## 目 录

## Unit 3   Common Pediatric Emergencies

## Unit 7　Common Traumas

　　　常见创伤　·················· 246

# Contents

目 录

# Unit 1

## Common Emergencies in Internal Medicine
## 内科常见急症

## Section 1　Coma
## 昏迷

### Conversation

　　Patient, male, 60 years old, suddenly lost consciousness at home. His family member called for emergency medical services and doctors arrived at the scene within 15 minutes.

　　病人,男性,60 岁,在家中突然昏迷,家属拨打了 120 急救电话,医生 15 分钟内到达现场。

　　**Doctor:** Hello, can you hear me? Can you tell me your name?

---

🔍 **Key Words and Phrases**

**emergency** [ɪˈmɜːdʒənsɪ] n. 紧急事件,紧急情况,非常时刻
**internal medicine** 内科医学
**coma** [ˈkəʊmə] n. <医> 昏迷
**consciousness** [ˈkɒnʃəsnəs] n. 意识,清醒状态

**医生**：您好，您能听到我说话吗，能告诉我您的名字吗？

*The patient is <u>unresponsive</u>. Doctor turns to the family member and asks questions.*

*病人没有回应。医生转向家属提问。*

**Doctor:** Hello, I'm Dr. Han. Would you please tell me what has happened to him?

**医生**：您好，我是韩医生。您能告诉我他怎么了吗？

**Patient's family member:** Yes, my father suddenly fell down when he was washing the dishes. We kept calling him, but he didn't respond.

**病人家属**：我父亲在洗碗的时候突然摔倒了。我们一直在喊他，但他没有反应。

**Doctor:** When did he fall down?

**医生**：他什么时候摔倒的？

**Patient's family member:** About 20 minutes ago.

**病人家属**：大约 20 分钟前。

**Doctor:** He didn't make any response to your calling, did he?

**医生**：他对你们的呼叫没有反应，对吗？

**Patient's family member:** No.

**病人家属**：是的。

**Doctor:** What has he eaten before going into coma?

**医生**：他在昏迷之前吃了什么？

**Patient's family member:** Only a bowl of <u>porridge</u>.

**病人家属**：只喝了一碗粥。

> **🔍 Key Words and Phrases**
>
> **unresponsive** [ˌʌnrɪˈspɒnsɪv] adj. 无答复的，反应迟钝的
>
> **porridge** [ˈpɒrɪdʒ] n. 粥，麦片粥，稀饭

**Doctor:** Did he have any discomfort before falling down, such as headache, dizziness, vomiting or numbness in hands and feet?

医生:他在摔倒之前是否有任何不适？比如头痛、头晕、呕吐或者手脚麻木等。

**Patient's family member:** No.

病人家属:没有。

**Doctor:** Did you hear his abnormal breathing sounds?

医生:您有听到他发出异常的呼吸音吗？

**Patient's family member:** No.

病人家属:没有。

**Doctor:** Has he ever had any head injuries or seizures?

医生:他有过头部受伤或者癫痫发作史吗？

**Patient's family member:** No.

病人家属:没有。

**Doctor:** Has he had any chronic diseases, such as hypertension, diabetes or cerebral infarction?

---

### 🔍 Key Words and Phrases

**discomfort** [dɪsˈkʌmfət] n. 不舒适, 不舒服, 不安;v. 使……不舒服, 使……不安

**dizziness** [ˈdɪzɪnəs] n. 头昏眼花

**vomiting** [ˈvɒmɪtɪŋ] n. 呕吐

**numbness** [nʌmnəs] n. 无感觉, 麻木

**abnormal** [æbˈnɔːml] adj. 不正常的, 异常的, 畸形的

**seizure** [ˈsiːʒə(r)] n.（癫痫）突然发作

**chronic diseases** <医> 慢性疾病

**hypertension** [ˌhaɪpəˈtenʃn] n. 高血压

**diabetes** [ˌdaɪəˈbiːtiːz] n. 糖尿病

**cerebral infarction** 脑梗死

医生：他是否有慢性疾病？比如高血压、糖尿病、脑梗死。

**Patient's family member:** He has suffered from hypertension and has been taking <u>antihypertensive</u> <u>medications</u>.

病人家属：他有高血压，一直在服用降压药。

**Doctor:** Has any of his family members ever had similar health condition?

医生：他的家族中有人曾有过类似的状况吗？

**Patient's family member:** I haven't heard about that.

病人家属：我没有听说过。

**Doctor:** Has he ever had operation?

医生：他有过手术史吗？

**Patient's family member:** No.

病人家属：没有。

**Doctor:** Thank you for your information! We will have basic examination on him.

医生：谢谢您提供的信息！我们马上给他做一些基础的检查。

*After the examination.*

*检查后。*

**Doctor:** Your father has gone into coma. Although he currently has normal <u>respiration</u>, <u>pupils</u>, <u>oxygen saturation</u> and

---

**Key Words and Phrases**

**antihypertensive** [ˈæntiːhɑɪpəˈtensɪv] adj. & n. 抗高血压的（药物）

**medication** [medɪˈkeɪʃn] n. 药物，敷药，施药

**pulse** [pʌls] n. 脉搏；v.（心脏）跳动，脉动，搏动

**respiration** [ˌrespəˈreɪʃn] n. 呼吸

**pupils** [ˈpjuːplz] n. 瞳孔

**oxygen saturation** 血氧饱和度

heart rate, his blood pressure is high. Moreover, he has reduced muscle strength in one limb. There are many causes for coma. According to his signs, he is more likely to have cerebrovascular accident. He needs further examination and treatment, so we must send him to the hospital as soon as possible.

医生：您父亲处于昏迷状态。虽然他目前呼吸、瞳孔、血氧饱和度和心率正常，但他血压高且一侧肢体肌力减退。造成昏迷的原因有很多，根据其体征判断，他很可能发生了脑血管意外，需要进一步检查和治疗，所以我们必须尽快把他送去医院。

**Patient's family member:** Does my father have cerebral infarction? Please treat him with vasodilators immediately.

病人家属：医生，我父亲是不是脑梗死了？请您赶紧用血管扩张药为他治疗。

**Doctor:** Cerebrovascular accident is divided into cerebral hemorrhage and cerebral infarction, which needs different treatments. We shouldn't blindly use vasodilators. He needs to have cranial CT or head MRI and other examinations to make a definite diagnosis.

---

### 🔍 Key Words and Phrases

**strength** [streŋθ] n. 体力，强度

**limb** [lɪm] n. 肢体

**cerebrovascular accident** 脑血管意外

**vasodilators** [ˌvɔsədaɪˈleɪtəz] n. <医> 血管扩张药

**cerebral hemorrhage** 脑出血

**cranial** [ˈkreɪnɪəl] adj. 头盖的，头盖形的

**diagnosis** [ˌdaɪəgˈnəʊsɪs] n. 诊断，判断

医生：脑血管意外分为脑出血和脑梗死，它们的治疗原则不一样，我们不能盲目使用血管扩张药。他需要进行头颅 CT 或者头部核磁共振等检查来明确诊断。

**Patient's family members:** Is there no treatment for the time being?

病人家属：目前不做治疗吗？

**Doctor:** We will establish the <u>intravenous</u> access and give him some <u>symptomatic treatments</u>, such as some medications to control the blood pressure and oxygen. In the <u>ambulance</u>, we will keep his airway open as well as <u>monitor</u> his breathing, pulse, blood pressure and oxygen saturation. If his vital signs <u>deteriorate</u> on the way, we will take <u>corresponding</u> measures to <u>stabilize</u> his condition.

医生：我们会给病人开放静脉通道并进行对症处理，比如注射一些药物控制血压和吸氧。在救护车上，我们会保持他的呼吸道通畅，监控呼吸、脉搏、血压和血氧饱和度。此外，如果在途中，他的生命体征恶化，我们会采取对应的救治措施稳定病情。

---

### 🔍 Key Words and Phrases

**intravenous** [ˌɪntrəˈviːnəs] adj. 进入静脉的，静脉注射的

**symptomatic treatment** 对症治疗，症状疗法

**ambulance** [ˈæmbjələns] n. 救护车

**monitor** [ˈmɒnɪtə(r)] v. 监控，监听

**deteriorate** [dɪˈtɪəriəreɪt] v. 恶化，变坏，衰退

**corresponding** [ˌkɒrəˈspɒndɪŋ] adj. 相应的，相关的；v. 符合

**stabilize** [ˈsteɪbəlaɪz] v.（使）稳定，（使）稳固，变得稳定

**Patient's family member:** Got it, thank you!

病人家属：明白了，谢谢。

## Useful Expressions

Did the coma start abruptly or gradually?

病人是突然昏迷还是缓慢发病？

Has the patient had any chronic diseases, such as diabetes, stroke or heart attack?

病人是否有慢性疾病？比如糖尿病、脑卒中、心脏病。

Has any of his / her family members ever had similar health condition?

他／她的家族中有人曾有过类似的状况吗？

Has he / she ever had operation?

他／她是否有过手术史？

Has the patient recently taken medications?

病人最近是否在服用药物？

Is the patient likely to have drug overdose?

病人是否有可能服药过量？

Is the patient likely to be poisoned?

病人是否有可能中毒？

What has the patient eaten before going into coma?

病人在昏迷前吃了什么食物？

---

🔍 **Key Words and Phrases**

**drug overdose** <医>（药）过量

**poisoned** ['pɔɪzənd] adj. 有毒的，中毒的

Did you hear his / her abnormal breathing sounds?

您有听到他 / 她发出异常的呼吸音吗?

Has the patient ever experienced a head injury?

病人头部是否受过伤?

Has the patient ever had a seizure?

病人有癫痫发作史吗?

Has the patient married or ever been pregnant? (To female)

病人是否有过婚孕史?（针对女性病人）

The patient is unresponsive, with a Glasgow Coma Scale score of […].

病人没有反应,格拉斯哥昏迷评分为［……］分。

The patient's airway is […], and he is breathing at the rate of […] breaths per minute.

病人的气道状态为［……］,呼吸频率为［……］次 /min。

The patient has a pulse of […] beats per minute and blood pressure of […] / […] mmHg.

病人的脉搏为［……］次 /min, 血压为［……］/［……］ mmHg。

We're going to transport him / her to the hospital for further evaluation and treatment.

我们将把他 / 她送到医院进行进一步评估和治疗。

---

Key Words and Phrases

**Glasgow Coma Scale** 格拉斯哥昏迷评分

**transport** [trænˈspɔːt] v. 运送,运输

# Section 2　Syncope
## 晕厥

## Conversation

**Patient, female, 39 years old, suddenly <u>fainted</u> at home. Her family member called for emergency medical services.**

病人,女性,39 岁,在家中突然晕倒,家属拨打了 120 急救电话。

**Doctor:** Hello, I'm Dr. Han. I was told that the patient had an <u>episode</u> of syncope. Can you tell me what has happened to her?

医生:您好,我是韩医生。我得知病人发生了晕厥。您能告诉我她怎么了吗?

**Patient's family member:** Yes, she suddenly passed out just now.

病人家属:是的,她刚才突然晕倒。

**Doctor:** What was she doing before she fainted? Did she have any discomfort, such as dizziness, <u>vertigo</u> or <u>palpitations</u>?

医生:她晕倒之前在做什么,有没有头晕、眩晕或心悸等

---

**🔍 Key Words and Phrases**

**syncope** [ˈsɪŋkəpi] n. 晕厥,昏厥
**faint** [ˈfeɪnt] adj. 微弱的,晕眩的;v. 晕倒;n. 昏厥
**episode** [ˈepɪsəʊd] n.(病症)发作期,一段经历
**vertigo** [ˈvɜːtɪɡəʊ] n. 眩晕,头晕
**palpitation** [ˌpælpɪˈteɪʃn] n. 心悸

不适？

**Patient's family member:** At the time, she was watching TV and feeling a little dizzy. So, she wanted to go to bed and lie down for a while. When she stood up, she suddenly fell on the floor and lost consciousness.

**病人家属:** 当时她在看电视,感觉有点头晕,想上床躺一会儿。当她站起来的时候,突然倒地,然后失去了意识。

**Doctor:** Got it. Did she have convulsion, foaming at the mouth or any other symptoms when she fainted?

**医生:** 明白。她晕厥时有抽搐、口吐白沫或者其他症状吗?

**Patient's family member:** She was pale and had cold sweat.

**病人家属:** 她脸色苍白、冒冷汗。

**Doctor:** Did she react to your calling?

**医生:** 她对你们的呼叫有反应吗?

**Patient's family member:** She didn't respond at the time, but she woke up after we gave her massage.

**病人家属:** 她当时没有反应,但我们给她按摩刺激后,她就醒来了。

**Doctor:** How long did the syncope last?

**医生:** 这次晕厥持续了多长时间?

**Patient's family member:** About 10 minutes.

**病人家属:** 大约 10 分钟。

*The doctor turns to the patient and asks questions.*

*医生转向病人提问。*

**Doctor:** How did you feel

---

🔍 **Key Words and Phrases**

**convulsion** [kən'vʌlʃn] n. <医> 抽搐

**foam** ['fəʊm] v. 起泡沫,吐白沫;n. 泡沫,泡沫材料

after waking up?

　　**医生：**您醒来后感觉怎么样？

**Patient:** A little dizzy and nauseous.

　　**病人：**有点头晕、恶心。

**Doctor:** Have you ever experienced similar syncope before?

　　**医生：**您以前有过类似的晕厥症状吗？

**Patient:** No, this is the first time.

　　**病人：**没有，这是第一次。

**Doctor:** Have you ever experienced chest pain or shortness of breath?

　　**医生：**您之前有过胸痛或呼吸困难吗？

**Patient:** No.

　　**病人：**没有。

**Doctor:** Have you had any physical examinations, such as an electrocardiogram (ECG), an electroencephalogram, or a skull X-ray?

　　**医生：**您做过体检吗？比如心电图、脑电图、头颅 X 线检查。

---

**🔍 Key Words and Phrases**

**nauseous** [ˈnɔ:ziəs] adj. 恶心的

**chest pain** 胸痛

**shortness of breath** 呼吸困难，气促

**electrocardiogram (ECG)** [ɪˌlektrəʊˈkɑ:diəʊgræm] n. 心电图，心电图仪器

**electroencephalogram** [ɪˌlektrəʊɪnˈsefələgræm] n. <医>脑电波，脑动电流图

**skull** [skʌl] n. 颅骨，头盖骨，脑袋

**Patient:** No.

病人：没有。

**Doctor:** Have you had any other diseases or taken any medications?

医生：您有没有其他疾病或服用什么药物?

**Patient:** No.

病人：没有。

**Doctor:** Thank you for the information! We will give you physical examination, electrocardiogram and blood glucose test.

医生：谢谢您提供的信息！我们会为您做体格检查、做心电图、测血糖。

**Patient:** OK.

病人：好的。

**Doctor:** You have a brief period of unconsciousness. Now, your blood pressure is low and breathing is a bit rapid. The temperature, pulse, oxygen saturation and electrocardiogram are basically normal. Cardiopulmonary auscultation shows no obvious abnormalities. The nurse will first give you oxygen to relieve your symptoms and at the same time obtain the intravenous access to replenish blood volume, etc. If your conditions get

---

🔍 **Key Words and Phrases**

**blood glucose** 血糖

**cardiopulmonary** [ˌkɑːdɪəʊˈpʌlmənərɪ] adj. <医> 心肺的

**auscultation** [ˌɔːskəlˈteɪʃn] n. 听诊

**abnormality** [ˌæbnɔːˈmælɪtɪ] n. (身体、行为等)不正常,反常

**replenish** [rɪˈplenɪʃ] v. 补充

worse, let us know immediately. If necessary, we will <u>administer</u> symptomatic treatment by intravenous medications to ease your conditions.

**医生**：您有一过性的意识障碍，现在血压偏低，呼吸有些急促。体温、脉搏、血氧饱和度、心电图基本正常。心肺部听诊未见明显异常。护士先给您吸氧缓解一下症状，同时开放静脉通道补充血容量等。如果您的症状加重，请立即告诉我们。必要时，我们会通过静脉注射药物来进行对症处理，缓解病情。

**Patient:** I see

**病人**：我明白了。

**Doctor:** There are many causes for syncope, including <u>vascular</u>, <u>cardiac</u> and cerebral factors. We need to send you to the hospital to find out the cause and give you further treatment.

**医生**：造成晕厥的原因很多，有血管性因素、心源性因素、脑源性因素，我们需要送您去医院，查找出晕厥的原因，并进行下一步治疗。

**Patient:** I'm feeling much better now. Do I still need to do the examinations?

**病人**：医生，我现在感觉好多了，还需要做检查吗？

**Doctor:** We will first conduct <u>auxiliary</u> examinations on your heart, blood vessels and blood to find out if there are any

---

### 🔍 Key Words and Phrases

**administer** [əd'mɪnɪstə(r)] v. 给予，施用（药物）

**vascular** ['væskjələ(r)] adj. 血管的，脉管的，含有血管的

**cardiac** ['kɑːdiæk] adj. 心脏（病）的，（胃的）贲门的

**auxiliary** [ɔːg'zɪliəri] adj. 辅助的

underlying medical conditions. If there is no abnormality, no treatment will be done for the time being. Next time, if you feel an episode of syncope coming on, such as feeling lightheaded, nauseous or having heart palpitations, please avoid standing up too quickly, especially after a long period of sitting or lying down.

医生：我们首先会对您进行心脏、血管、血液方面的辅助检查，了解您是否存在潜在的疾病。如果您身体没有异常，就暂时不做治疗。以后您如有预感要晕厥，比如感到头昏眼花、恶心或者心悸，请避免过快地站起来，尤其是在久坐或久卧之后。

**Patient:** OK, that sounds reasonable.

病人：好的，有道理。

## Useful Expressions

When did the patient pass out?

病人是什么时候晕倒的？

How long did it last?

持续了多长时间？

Did the patient have any discomfort before the syncope, such as dizziness, vertigo or palpitations?

病人在昏厥前有头晕、眩晕或心悸等不适吗？

Did the patient have convulsion, foaming at the mouth or any other symptoms when he / she fainted?

病人晕厥时有抽搐、口吐白沫或者其他症状吗？

Do you still remember what had happened before the patient

| Key Words and Phrases |
| --- |
| **underlying** [ˌʌndəˈlaɪɪŋ] adj. 基础的, 潜在的, 含蓄的, 表面下的, 下层的 |

passed out?

您还记得病人在晕厥前发生了什么事吗?

Has the patient ever experienced similar episodes before that?

病人以前是否有过类似的发作?

Has the patient ever had allergies or other diseases?

病人有过敏或其他疾病吗?

Has the patient had any physical examinations, such as an electrocardiogram, an electroencephalogram, or a skull X-ray?

病人做过体检吗? 比如心电图、脑电图、头颅 X 线检查。

There are many causes for syncope, including vascular, cardiac and cerebral factors.

造成晕厥的原因很多,有血管性因素、心源性因素、脑源性因素。

We will first conduct auxiliary examinations on your heart, blood vessels and blood to find out if there are any underlying medical conditions.

我们首先会对您进行心脏、血管、血液方面的辅助检查,了解您是否存在潜在的疾病。

## Section 3　Tic
## 抽搐

### Conversation

**Patient, female, 17 years old, has been experiencing tics for half an hour and her family**

🔍 **Key Words and Phrases**

**tic** [tɪk] n.(尤指面部或头部肌肉的)抽搐,痉挛

member called for emergency medical services.

病人,女性,17 岁,出现抽搐半小时,家属拨打了 120 急救电话。

**Doctor:** Hi, I'm Dr. Han. I was told that the patient has been experiencing tics. Can you tell me something more about her symptoms?

医生:您好,我是韩医生。我得知病人有抽搐症状。关于她的症状,您能告诉我更多的信息吗?

**Patient's family member:** Yes, she has rapid, recurring contractions in group of muscles like this, out of control.

病人家属:好的,她的肌肉群快速、反复收缩,就像这样,不受控制。

**Doctor:** When did it start?

医生:什么时候开始的?

**Patient's family member:** Half an hour ago.

病人家属:半小时前。

**Doctor:** Is it a continuous tonic convulsion or an intermittent clonic convulsion?

医生:是持续性强直性抽搐还是间歇性阵挛性抽搐?

---

**Q　Key Words and Phrases**

**contraction** [kən'trækʃən] n. 收缩,(分娩时)子宫收缩

**continuous** [kən'tɪnjuəs] adj. 连续不断的,没有间隔的

**tonic convulsion** < 医 > 强直性抽搐

**intermittent** [ˌɪntə'mɪtənt] adj. 间歇的,断断续续的

**clonic convulsion** 阵挛性惊厥,抽搐

**Patient's family member:** Intermittent one.

病人家属:间歇性的。

**Doctor:** How long does it last?

医生:持续了多长时间?

**Patient's family member:** About 30 minutes.

病人家属:大约 30 分钟。

**Doctor:** Was she foaming at the mouth, <u>incontinent</u> or unconscious during the attack?

医生:抽搐发作时,她是否有口吐白沫、大小便失禁以及失去意识的症状?

**Patient's family member:** No.

病人家属:没有。

**Doctor:** Did she respond to your calls when she had an attack?

医生:症状发作时,她对你们的呼叫有反应吗?

**Patient's family member:** Occasionally.

病人家属:偶尔有。

**Doctor:** Has she ever had these symptoms before?

医生:她既往有过这种症状吗?

**Patient's family member:** Once.

病人家属:以前有过一次。

**Doctor:** When did she have first tic?

医生:她第一次抽搐发作是什么时候?

**Patient's family member:**
A few months ago.

病人家属:几个月前。

**Doctor:** Has she had a lot

**Q  Key Words and Phrases**

**incontinent** [ɪnˈkɒntɪnənt] adj.
(大小便)失禁的,不能自制的

· 17 ·

of mood swings lately? Were there any obvious triggers like stress or anxiety?

**医生:** 她最近情绪波动大吗,抽搐发作有明显的诱因吗? 比如压力或焦虑。

**Patient's family member:** Yes, she has too much academic pressure. She complained about feeling tense before this and last attack.

**病人家属:** 是的,她觉得学习压力很大,上次和这次发作前她都说感到紧张。

**Doctor:** Has she ever seen a doctor?

**医生:** 她之前看过医生吗?

**Patient's family member:** No, she recovered a few minutes later last time. And last attack was localized and she was conscious, nothing like today.

**病人家属:** 没有,她上次发作了几分钟就好了,而且是局部的,意识清醒,跟今天完全不一样。

**Doctor:** Has she had any cardiovascular, cerebrovascular, psychiatric, metabolic disorders or other diseases?

---

### 🔍 Key Words and Phrases

**mood swings** 情绪波动

**trigger** ['trɪgə] n. 诱因;v. 引发

**localized** ['ləʊkəlaɪzd] adj. 局限性的,地区的

**cardiovascular** [ˌkɑ:diəʊˈvæskjələ(r)] adj. 心血管的

**cerebrovascular** [ˌserəbrəʊˈvæskjələ] adj. 脑血管的

**psychiatric** [ˌsaɪkiˈætrɪk] adj. 精神病学的,精神病治疗的

**metabolic** [ˌmetəˈbɒlɪk] adj. 新陈代谢的

医生:她是否有心脑血管疾病、精神疾病、代谢障碍或者其他疾病?

**Patient's family member:** No.

病人家属:没有。

**Doctor:** Has she had any head injuries?

医生:她的头部受过伤吗?

**Patient's family member:** No.

病人家属:没有。

**Doctor:** Has she been taking medications?

医生:她是否在服用药物?

**Patient's family member:** No.

病人家属:没有。

**Doctor:** What symptoms did she have after tic?

医生:抽搐停止后她有什么症状?

**Patient's family member:** She seemed to have no obvious symptoms.

病人家属:好像没有明显症状。

**Doctor:** Has anyone in the family ever had tic or neurological disorders?

医生:家族中有人有过抽搐或神经系统疾病吗?

**Patient's family member:** No.

病人家属:没有。

*Doctor turns to the patient and asks questions.*

*医生转向病人提问。*

**Doctor:** How do you

---

**Key Words and Phrases**

**neurological** [ˌnjʊərəˈlɒdʒɪkl] adj.
神经学的,神经病学的

feel now?

医生：您现在感觉怎样？

Patient: Dizzy, fatigue and fearful.

病人：头晕、乏力并且感到恐惧。

Doctor: I see. Is it OK to give you physical and auxiliary examination?

医生：我明白了。现在是否可以对您进行体格检查和辅助检查呢？

Patient: Yes.

病人：可以。

Doctor: Based on the medical history, symptoms and signs, your tic may be related to stress, anxiety or neurological disorders. Please try to relax.

医生：根据病史、症状和体征判断，您的抽搐可能与压力、焦虑或者神经系统疾病有关。请尽量放松！

Patient: OK.

病人：好。

Doctor: Don't be nervous! We need to send you to the hospital for further examination and evaluation to rule out other causes. OK?

医生：别紧张。我们需要将您送往医院，进行进一步检查和评估以排除其他病因，可以吗？

Patient: OK.

病人：行。

Doctor: We will keep your airway open and monitor your

> 🔍 **Key Words and Phrases**
>
> **rule out** 排除……的可能性

breathing, pulse, blood pressure and oxygen saturation in the ambulance. If necessary, we will also administer some medications to <u>sedate</u> and relieve your tic.

**医生**：我们在救护车上会保持您的呼吸道通畅，监控呼吸、脉搏、血压和血氧饱和度。必要时，我们还会使用一些药物来镇静和缓解抽搐。

**Patient:** OK, thanks.

**病人**：好的，谢谢。

## Useful Expressions

When did the patient start to have a tic?

病人什么时候开始抽搐的？

How long did it last?

持续了多长时间？

Were there any obvious triggers for tic?

是否有明显的诱因导致抽搐？

Was the tic generalized or localized?

是全身性抽搐还是局部性抽搐？

Is it a continuous tonic convulsion or an intermittent clonic convulsion?

是持续性强直性抽搐还是间歇性阵挛性抽搐？

Was the patient foaming at the mouth, incontinent or unconscious when he / she had a tic?

---

**Q Key Words and Phrases**

**sedate** [sɪˈdeɪt] v. 使镇静，给……服镇静剂；adj. 安静的，镇静的

病人抽搐发作时,是否有口吐白沫、大小便失禁以及失去意识的症状?

Has the patient ever had cardiovascular or cerebrovascular diseases?

病人是否心、脑血管疾病?

Has the patient ever had a head injury?

病人的头部受过伤吗?

Has the patient been taking medications?

病人是否在服用药物?

Has the patient had a lot of mood swings lately? Are there any obvious triggers like stress or anxiety?

病人最近情绪波动大吗,抽搐发作有明显的诱因吗? 比如压力或焦虑。

Did the tic interfere with his / her daily life and activities?

抽搐影响他 / 她的日常生活和活动吗?

Has anyone in patient's family ever had a tic or neurological diseases?

病人家族中有人曾有过抽搐或神经系统疾病吗?

Based on the medical history, symptoms and signs, the patient's tic may be related to stress, anxiety or neurological disorders. Please try to relax.

根据病史、症状和体征判断,病人的抽搐可能与压力、焦虑或者神经系统疾病有关。请尽量放松。

# Section 4　Acute Cerebrovascular Disease
# 急性脑血管病

## Conversation

Patient, female, 65 years old, suddenly had a severe headache and felt dizzy at home. A few minutes later, she had slurred speech and started having trouble moving her left arm and leg. Her family member called for emergency medical services.

病人，女性，65 岁，在家中突然出现了剧烈头痛和眩晕。几分钟后，她说话变得含糊不清，左侧肢体开始行动不便，家属拨打了 120 急救电话。

**Doctor:** Can you tell me what has happened to her?

医生：您能告诉我她怎么了吗?

**Patient's family member:** Yes, when we were talking happily, my mother suddenly complained of a severe headache and feeling dizzy. So, I helped her lie down. But a few minutes later, she couldn't speak clearly and she also vomited. Then I noticed that her left arm and leg were so stiff that she couldn't move freely.

---

### 🔍 Key Words and Phrases

acute cerebrovascular disease 急性脑血管病

slurred [slə:d] adj. 含糊的，难以听见（或理解）的

stiff [stɪf] adj. 严厉的，僵硬的，坚硬的，呆板的，拘谨的

**病人家属：**好的，当时我们聊天聊得很开心，我的母亲突然说她头很痛、很晕，我就扶她躺下。但几分钟后，她开始言语不清，还呕吐了。然后，我发现她的左侧肢体僵硬得无法自由活动了。

*Doctor turns to the patient and asks questions, but she can't answer clearly, so the doctor turns back to the family member again.*

医生转向病人提问，但她回答不清，医生再次转向家属提问。

**Doctor:** When did she start to have these symptoms?

**医生：**她什么时候开始发病的？

**Patient's family member:** About half an hour ago.

**病人家属：**大约半小时前。

**Doctor:** Did she show these symptoms suddenly or progressively?

**医生：**这些症状是突然出现的还是逐渐出现的？

**Patient's family member:** Suddenly.

**病人家属：**是突然出现的。

**Doctor:** Has she ever fainted or gone into a coma?

**医生：**她有晕厥或者昏迷吗？

**Patient's family member:** No.

**病人家属：**没有。

**Doctor:** Was she incontinent?

**医生：**她是否有大小便失禁？

**Patient's family member:** Yes.

**病人家属：**是的。

> 🔍 **Key Words and Phrases**
>
> **progressively** [prə'gresɪvli] adv.
> 逐步，前进地，日益增加地

**Doctor:** Has she had high blood pressure, diabetes or high cholesterol?

医生：她是否有高血压、糖尿病或高胆固醇？

**Patient's family member:** Yes, she has had high blood pressure and high cholesterol.

病人家属：是的，她有高血压，胆固醇也高。

**Doctor:** Has she ever had heart problems?

医生：她之前有过心脏方面的疾病吗？

**Patient's family member:** She was diagnosed with coronary heart disease five years ago, so she has been taking medications regularly. Her blood pressure and coronary heart disease have been well controlled.

病人家属：她 5 年前被诊断为冠心病，所以在按时吃药，她的血压和冠心病一直控制得很好。

**Doctor:** Has she ever had drug allergies?

医生：她有药物过敏吗？

**Patient's family member:** I am not sure.

病人家属：我不清楚。

**Doctor:** We need to test her blood sugar and neurological system.

医生：我们需要对她的血糖以及神经系统进行检查。

---

**🔍 Key Words and Phrases**

**cholesterol** [kə'lestərɒl] n. 胆固醇

**diagnose** ['daiəgnəuz] v. 诊断

**coronary heart disease** 冠状动脉性心脏病，冠心病

**Patient's family member:** OK.

病人家属：好的。

**Doctor:** Her blood pressure and blood sugar are high, and she had hemiplegia, too. All these may be related to acute cerebrovascular disease (ACVD). Time is critical for acute cerebrovascular disease patient, and early treatment can make a big difference. So, we need to send her to the hospital as soon as possible for further examination and treatment.

医生：她血压、血糖都高，且有肢体偏瘫。这些症状可能跟急性脑血管病有关。对于这类疾病的病人来说，时间节点非常关键，早期治疗起着重要的作用。所以我们需要尽快送她去医院，接受进一步的检查和治疗。

**Patient's family member:** Is it life-threatening?

病人家属：她有生命危险吗？

**Doctor:** We are now using medications to control her blood pressure and blood sugar as well as try to keep her condition stable. In the ambulance, if there is a change in her condition, we will give her necessary emergency treatment.

医生：我们正在用药物控制她的血压和血糖，尽量保证病情稳定。在救护车上，如果她的病情有变化，我们会对她采取必要的急救措施。

**Patient's family member:** What treatments are needed?

### Key Words and Phrases

**hemiplegia** [ˌhemɪˈpliːdʒɪə] n. 偏瘫，半身麻痹，半身不遂

**critical** [ˈkrɪtɪkl] adj. 关键的，(病情)严重的

**life-threatening** [laɪf ˈθretnɪŋ] adj. 威胁生命的

**病人家属**:她一般要做哪些治疗?

**Doctor:** We will perform a thorough evaluation. If she has cerebral infarction, we can inject her with medications to dissolve blood clots or remove blood clots by surgery in the golden hour. If she has cerebral hemorrhage, we will determine surgical approach based on the location and the amount of bleeding.

**医生**:我们将进行全面评估。如果她是脑梗死,在时间窗内,我们可以通过注射药物来溶解血栓或通过手术清除血栓;如果她是脑出血,我们会根据出血位置和出血量决定手术方式。

**Patient's family member:** Please!

**病人家属**:拜托你们了!

## Useful Expressions

When did these symptoms start?

这些症状是什么时候开始的?

How long did it last?

持续了多长时间?

Has the patient had headaches, dizziness or vomiting?

病人有头痛、头晕、呕吐症状吗?

Has the patient had slurred speech or weak limb?

病人是否有言语不清、肢体无力症状?

---

### 🔍 Key Words and Phrases

**inject** [ɪnˈdʒekt] v.(给……)注射(药物等)

**dissolve** [dɪˈzɒlv] v.(使)溶解,解除,终止,消除

**clot** [klɒt] n. 凝块,血块;v. 凝固

**surgery** [ˈsɜːdʒəri] n. 外科手术

Did he/she show these symptoms suddenly or progressively?

这些症状是突然出现还是逐渐出现的？

Has the patient had hypertension, diabetes or high cholesterol?

病人是否有高血压、糖尿病或高胆固醇？

Has the patient had a stroke or heart attack before?

病人之前是否有过脑卒中或心脏病？

Has the patient ever had drug allergies?

病人有药物过敏吗？

We need to test the patient's blood sugar levels and nervous system.

我们需要对病人的血糖水平以及神经系统进行检查。

We will administer medications to manage the patient's blood pressure.

我们将用药物来控制病人的血压。

Time is critical for acute cerebrovascular disease patient, and early treatment can make a big difference.

对于急性脑血管病的病人而言，时间节点非常关键，早期治疗起着重要的作用。

If he / she has cerebral infarction, we can inject medications to dissolve blood clots or remove blood clots by surgery in the golden hour.

如果他 / 她是脑梗死，在时间窗内，我们可以通过注射药物来溶解血栓或通过手术清除血栓。

If he / she has cerebral hemorrhage, we will determine surgical approach based on the location and the amount of bleeding.

如果他 / 她是脑出血，我们会根据出血位置和出血量决定手术方式。

# Section 5   Hypoglycemia
# 低血糖症

## Conversation

**Patient, male, 35 years old, had consciousness disorder after repeatedly experiencing fatigue, palpitations and hand tremors for 1 hour. His family member called for emergency medical services.**

病人,男性,35 岁,在反复乏力、心悸、手抖 1 小时后出现意识障碍,家属拨打了 120 急救电话。

**Doctor:** Hello, I'm Dr. Han. What's the matter with your family?

医生:您好,我是韩医生。您家人怎么了?

**Patient's family member:** This morning, my husband was feeling unwell with palpitations, hand trembling and extreme fatigue. So, we suggested him to rest for a while. However, an hour later, he suddenly had confusion and began to speak unclearly.

病人家属:我丈夫今天早上就开始感觉不舒服,心悸、手

---

🔍 **Key Words and Phrases**

**hypoglycemia** [ˌhaɪpəʊglaɪˈsiːmɪə] n. 血糖过低,低血糖症

**fatigue** [fəˈtiːg] n. 疲劳,厌倦

**tremor** [ˈtremə(r)] n. 震颤,战栗

**confusion** [kənˈfjuːʒn] n. 意识模糊,混淆

抖,还非常乏力。我们建议他休息一下。但是一个小时后,他突然意识模糊,言语不清了。

**Doctor:** Could he wake up when you called him?

医生:您呼叫他时,他能否醒过来?

**Patient's family member:** He could wake up, but he went back to sleep again soon.

病人家属:他可以醒来,但是很快又会睡过去。

**Doctor:** Could he answer questions correctly?

医生:他能正确回答问题吗?

**Patient's family member:** Not very accurately.

病人家属:不是很准确。

**Doctor:** When did he start having these symptoms?

医生:他什么时候开始有这些症状的?

**Patient's family member:** About an hour ago, but these symptoms have been recurring for the past month.

病人家属:大约 1 小时前,但这个月来这些症状反复发生。

**Doctor:** Oh, how often?

医生:哦,多久发生一次?

**Patient's family member:** 2 or 3 times a week.

病人家属:一周两三次。

**Doctor:** Did he have a low body temperature or rapid heartbeat at the onset of the illness?

医生:他发病的时候是否有体温降低、心跳过快的症状?

**Patient's family member:** Yes, he did.

| 🔍 **Key Words and Phrases** |
| --- |
| **heartbeat** [ˈhɑːtbiːt] n. 心跳,心搏 |
| **onset** [ˈɒnset] n. <医> 发病,攻击,袭击 |

**病人家属**:是的。

**Doctor:** Has he had any other symptoms recently other than those just mentioned?

**医生**:除了刚才提到的症状外,他最近还有别的不舒服吗?

**Patient's family member:** He did mention that he has trouble concentrating lately.

**病人家属**:他有提到过,最近很难集中注意力。

**Doctor:** What's his dietary habits? Does he eat regularly?

**医生**:他的饮食习惯怎么样,有按时吃饭吗?

**Patient's family member:** Yes, he eats regularly and keeps on exercises, too.

**病人家属**:他按时吃饭,还坚持锻炼。

**Doctor:** Has he had hyperthyroidism or similar conditions?

**医生**:他有甲状腺功能亢进或类似疾病吗?

**Patient's family member:** No.

**病人家属**:没有。

**Doctor:** Has he had diabetes, hypertension, heart or kidney diseases?

**医生**:他有糖尿病、高血压、心脏或者肾脏疾病吗?

**Patient's family member:** Yes, he was diagnosed with type 1

---

🔍 **Key Words and Phrases**

**mention** ['menʃn] v. 提到,说起

**concentrate** ['kɒnsntreɪt] v. 专心于,注意,集中,聚集

**dietary** ['daɪətərɪ] adj. 饮食的,膳食中的;n. 规定的食物

**hyperthyroidism** [ˌhaɪpəˈθaɪrɔɪdɪzəm] n. 甲状腺功能亢进

**kidney** ['kɪdni] n. 肾,肾脏

diabetes.

**病人家属**：是的,他被确诊为 1 型糖尿病。

**Doctor:** Has he been taking the diabetes medication as prescribed?

**医生**：他有没有按照处方服用糖尿病治疗药物?

**Patient's family member:** Yes.

**病人家属**：是的。

**Doctor:** What is his usual blood sugar?

**医生**：他的血糖值通常是多少?

**Patient's family member:** No record on purpose.

**病人家属**：没有特意记录。

**Doctor:** Has he recently had infection or trauma?

**医生**：他最近有感染或外伤吗?

**Patient's family member:** No.

**病人家属**：没有。

**Doctor:** OK, how many hours has it been since he ate last time?

**医生**：好的,距离他上一次吃东西有几个小时了?

**Patient's family member:** It's been a few hours. He hasn't had anything since breakfast.

**病人家属**：已经几个小时了。早餐之后,他就没再吃东西了。

**Doctor:** We need to give him a relevant physical examination.

**医生**：我们需要为他进行相关的体格检查。

> 🔍 **Key Words and Phrases**
>
> **infection** [ɪnˈfekʃn] n. < 医 > 传染,感染,传染病
>
> **trauma** [ˈtrɔːmə] n. 损伤,创伤(由心理创伤造成精神上的异常)

**Patient's family member:** OK.

病人家属：好的。

**Doctor:** The nurse has just given him a quick check. His blood pressure, pulse, oxygen saturation and heart rate are normal, but his temperature is relatively low and his blood sugar is very low. These symptoms may be related to hypoglycemia. We will give him some <u>glucose</u> to raise his blood sugar levels.

医生：护士刚才给他进行了快速检查，他的血压、脉搏、血氧饱和度和心率都正常，但是体温偏低，血糖非常低。这些症状可能跟低血糖有关。我们会为他提供一些葡萄糖来提高他的血糖水平。

**Patient's family member:** Is his condition serious? He hasn't regained consciousness yet.

病人家属：他的病情严重吗？他现在还没有恢复意识呢。

**Doctor:** Confusion is a kind of consciousness disorder with many causes, so we have to send him to the hospital as soon as possible for further examination and treatment.

医生：意识模糊属于意识障碍的一种，病因有多种，我们要尽快送他去医院进行进一步检查和治疗。

**Patient's family member:** Is it life-threatening?

病人家属：他有生命危险吗？

**Doctor:** The nurse has already given him intravenous glucose to quickly raise his blood sugar levels. In the ambulance, we'll continue to monitor his vital signs and have appropriate treatment if

> 🔍 **Key Words and Phrases**
>
> **glucose** [ˈgluːkəʊs] n. < 化 >
> 葡萄糖，右旋糖

necessary.

医生：护士已经对他进行静脉注射葡萄糖来快速提升他的血糖水平。在救护车上，我们会继续监控他的生命体征，必要时会采取相应的救治措施。

**Patient's family member:** OK, as soon as possible.

病人家属：好的，那就尽快吧。

## Useful Expressions

Did the patient have low body temperature or rapid heartbeat at the onset of the illness?

病人在发病的时候是否有体温降低、心跳过快症状？

Has the patient had diabetes, hypertension, heart or kidney diseases?

病人有糖尿病、高血压、心脏或者肾脏疾病吗？

Has the patient ever had hypoglycemia?

病人以前有过低血糖吗？

Has the patient been taking the diabetes medication as prescribed?

病人有没有按照医生的建议服用糖尿病治疗药物？

What is the patient's usual blood sugar?

病人的血糖值通常是多少？

We need to examine the patient's blood sugar levels to determine the cause.

我们要检查病人的血糖水平以确定病因。

We'll give the patient some glucose to raise his / her blood sugar levels.

我们会为病人提供一些葡萄糖来提高他／她的血糖水平。

Remember to eat regularly and have medications as prescribed to maintain the blood sugar levels.

记得按时进食并遵照处方服用药物以稳定血糖水平。

## Section 6　Diabetic Ketoacidosis
### 糖尿病酮症酸中毒

## Conversation

**Patient, male, 50 years old, had experienced short breath, abdominal pain, dizziness and headache one day ago. Half an hour ago, he had consciousness disorder and his family member called for emergency medical services.**

病人，男性，50 岁，一天前开始出现气促、腹痛、头晕、头痛症状。半小时前，他出现意识障碍，家属拨打了 120 急救电话。

**Doctor:** Hello, I'm Dr. Han. Can you tell me your name?

医生：您好，我是韩医生。您能告诉我您的名字吗？

*Patient is unresponsive, and doctor turns to the family member.*

*病人没有反应，医生转向家属。*

**Doctor:** What is the matter with him?

医生：他怎么了？

---

🔍 **Key Words and Phrases**

**diabetic ketoacidosis** 糖尿病酮症酸中毒
**abdominal pain** 腹痛，腹部疼痛

**Patient's family member:** My husband seems to have lost consciousness.

病人家属:我丈夫好像失去意识了。

**Doctor:** When did you notice his unconsciousness?

医生:您是什么时候发现他失去意识的?

**Patient's family member:** About half an hour ago.

病人家属:大约半小时前。

**Doctor:** Besides being unconscious, did he have any other symptoms such as loss of control of his arms and legs, incontinence or foaming at the mouth?

医生:他除了失去意识外,有没有肢体失控、大小便失禁、口吐白沫等症状?

**Patient's family member:** No, he didn't.

病人家属:没有。

**Doctor:** Did he have hemiplegia?

医生:他有肢体偏瘫吗?

**Patient's family member:** No.

病人家属:没有

**Doctor:** What was he doing before he lost consciousness?

医生:在失去意识之前,他在做什么?

**Patient's family member:** Nothing, just lying in bed.

病人家属:没做什么,只是躺在床上。

**Doctor:** Before losing consciousness, has he had any symptoms recently?

医生:失去意识之前,最近他有什么症状吗?

**Patient's family member:** He had felt weak, dizzy and poor appetite last week. Yesterday he started having nausea, headache, shortness of breath and abdominal pain.

**病人家属：**他上周觉得乏力、头晕、没胃口，昨天开始恶心、头痛、气短和腹痛。

**Doctor:** Has he also had thirst, frequent urination, blurred vision or drowsiness?

**医生：**他有口渴、尿频、视物模糊、嗜睡症状吗？

**Patient's family member:** Yes. He recently has had a dry mouth, drunk a lot of water, urinated more often than before and sometimes had blurred vision.

**病人家属：**是的。他最近口干，喝了很多水，小便次数也比之前多，有时候说看东西不清楚。

**Doctor:** Has he been under stress or exposed to toxic substances recently?

**医生：**他最近是否压力大或者接触到有毒物质？

**Patient's family member:** I haven't heard about that.

**病人家属：**我没有听说。

**Doctor:** Has he had diabetes, hypertension or cardiovascular diseases?

---

🔍 **Key Words and Phrases**

**thirst** [θɜːst] n.（口）渴，干渴
**frequent urination** 尿频
**blurred vision** 视物模糊，视力障碍
**drowsiness** [ˈdraʊzɪnəs] n. 睡意，嗜睡
**be exposed to** 暴露于，暴露在，面临
**toxic substance** 有毒物质

**医生**：他患有糖尿病、高血压或者心血管疾病吗？

**Patient's family member:** He has had <u>hyperglycemia</u> and hypertension, but no cardiovascular diseases.

**病人家属**：他患有高血糖症和高血压，但没有心血管疾病。

**Doctor:** Which type of diabetes has he been diagnosed?

**医生**：他患有哪个类型的糖尿病？

**Patient's family member:** Type 2.

**病人家属**：2 型。

**Doctor:** When did he start having hypertension and hyperglycemia?

**医生**：他什么时候开始患有高血压和高血糖症的？

**Patient's family member:** About 7 years ago.

**病人家属**：大约 7 年前。

**Doctor:** Has he been monitoring his blood sugar or hypertension according to his doctor's requirements?

**医生**：他有按照医生的要求监测血糖和血压吗？

**Patient's family member:** His blood pressure has been well controlled.

**病人家属**：他的血压控制得很好。

**Doctor:** Has he used <u>insulin</u> on time lately?

**医生**：他最近有按时用胰岛素吗？

**Patient's family member:** No, he has run out of insulin in the last few days.

**病人家属**：没有，他的胰岛素几天前用完了。

**Doctor:** Has he had any

> **Key Words and Phrases**
>
> **hyperglycemia** [ˌhaɪpəglaɪˈsiːmɪə]
> n. 多糖症，高血糖症
> **insulin** [ˈɪnsjəlɪn] n. 胰岛素

lung or infectious diseases?

医生:他有过肺部或者感染类疾病吗?

**Patient's family member:** Yes, he has recently had urinary tract infection.

病人家属:是的,他最近尿路感染了。

**Doctor:** I see. These symptoms could be related to hyperglycemia. Let's start by testing his blood sugar and vital signs as well as giving him physical examination.

医生:我明白了。这些症状可能跟高血糖有关。我们先给他测一下血糖、生命体征,并对他进行体格检查。

*After the quick examination.*

*在快速检查后。*

**Doctor:** His temperature and blood pressure are low, but his heart rate is fast and his blood sugar is extremely high. First, we will inject him with moderate insulin and other medications to relieve his symptoms. At the same time, we send him to the hospital as soon as possible for further examination and treatment.

医生:他的体温和血压低,但心率快,血糖非常高。我们先为他注射适量的胰岛素及其他药物来缓解病情。同时,尽快把他送去医院,进行进一步的检查和治疗。

---

🔍 **Key Words and Phrases**

**infectious** [ɪnˈfekʃəs] adj. 传染的,有传染性的,易传染的

**urinary tract infection** 尿路感染

**moderate** [ˈmɒdərət] adj. 适度的,中等的,稳健的,温和的;v. 使和缓

## Useful Expressions

Has the patient had diabetes? Which type?

病人有糖尿病吗,是哪个类型?

Has the patient had diabetes, hypertension or cardiovascular diseases?

病人有糖尿病、高血压或心血管疾病吗?

Has the patient been monitoring his blood sugar according to the doctor's requirement?

病人有按照医生的要求监测血糖吗?

Has the patient been experiencing any other symptoms, such as increased thirst, frequent urination, blurred vision or fatigue?

病人有口渴、尿频、视物模糊或乏力等其他症状吗?

Has the patient had any recent lung, urinary tract or other infections?

病人最近有肺部、尿路或者其他感染吗?

It's important to regularly monitor the blood sugar levels to prevent complications.

为了预防并发症,定期监测血糖水平很重要。

We need to adjust insulin and other medications dosage to better manage the blood sugar levels.

我们需要调整胰岛素及其他药物的剂量以更好地控制血糖

---

🔍 **Key Words and Phrases**

**complication** [ˌkɒmplɪˈkeɪʃən] n. <医> 并发症

**dosage** [ˈdəʊsɪdʒ] n. (药物等的) 剂量,用量

水平。

We need to perform a <u>glycosylated hemoglobin test</u> to better understand his / her blood sugar levels during this period.

我们需要进行糖化血红蛋白测试,以更好地了解他 / 她这段时间的血糖水平。

The patient's blood sugar levels are extremely high, so he / she needs to be <u>hospitalized</u> for further treatment and monitoring.

病人血糖非常高,他 / 她需要住院以进行进一步治疗和监测。

It's important to stay <u>hydrated</u>, so we're going to give him / her <u>fluids</u>.

保持充足水分很重要,所以我们将为他 / 她输液。

## Section 7　Acute Headache
## 急性头痛

## Conversation

**Patient, male, 46 years old, suddenly experienced severe headache. He was conscious and called for emergency medical services.**

---

🔍 **Key Words and Phrases**

**glycosylated hemoglobin test** 糖化血红蛋白测试

**hospitalize** [ˈhɒspɪtəlaɪz] v. 送……住院,使留医

**hydrated** [ˈhaɪdreɪtɪd] adj. 含水的,与水结合的

**fluid** [ˈfluːɪd] n. 液体,流体

---

病人,男性,46 岁,突发头部剧痛,意识清醒,自行拨打了 120 急救电话。

**Doctor:** Hello, I am a paramedic. What's the matter with you?

医生:您好,我是急救医生。您哪里不舒服?

**Patient:** I suddenly had a severe headache just now and still feel dizzy now.

病人:我刚才突然头痛得厉害,现在依然头晕眼花的。

**Doctor:** When did it occur? Have you ever had the similar experience before?

医生:什么时候开始的,您之前有过相似的经历吗?

**Patient:** About 30 minutes ago. I have never had such a severe headache before.

病人:大约 30 分钟前开始的,我之前从来没有这么剧烈的头痛经历。

**Doctor:** Any nausea or vomiting?

医生:有恶心、呕吐吗?

**Patient:** I vomited 2 times and felt better after that. But I still feel weak and dizzy now.

病人:我呕吐了 2 次,吐后感觉好点,但现在仍感觉虚弱、头晕。

---

🔍 **Key Words and Phrases**

**paramedic** [ˌpærəˈmedɪk] n. <美> 参与急救的医生,护理人员,医务辅助人员

**occur** [əˈkɜː(r)] v. 发生,存在于

**Doctor:** Did you have <u>blackout</u>, double vision or the feeling of objects <u>spinning</u> around you?

医生：您有眼前发黑、重影或者物体旋转感吗？

**Patient:** No.

病人：没有。

**Doctor:** Did you have <u>chest tightness</u>, chest pain or other symptoms?

医生：您有胸闷、胸痛或其他症状吗？

**Patient:** No.

病人：没感觉。

**Doctor:** Have you had any chronic diseases such as high blood pressure or diabetes?

医生：您既往有高血压、糖尿病等慢性疾病吗？

**Patient:** Yes. I have had hypertension for 10 years.

病人：是的，我患高血压 10 年了。

**Doctor:** Have you taken oral antihypertensive medication regularly? How has your blood pressure been?

医生：您有定期口服降压药物吗，血压控制得如何？

**Patient:** I have taken medication every day. My blood pressure has been a little high lately probably due to lack of sleep.

病人：我每天都吃药，最近可能是因为睡眠不足，血压有点高。

**Doctor:** Have you had limb numbness and fatigue?

医生：您有四肢麻木、乏

---

**Q  Key Words and Phrases**

**blackout** [ˈblækaʊt] n. 暂时失去知觉

**spin** [ˈspɪn] v. 使……旋转

**chest tightness** <医> 胸部紧迫感，胸闷

力吗?

**Patient:** Not obvious.

病人:这种感觉不明显。

**Doctor:** You have a sudden onset headache and high blood pressure, so let me perform a simple neurological examination on you.

医生:您头痛突然发作,而且有高血压病史,我先给您做一个简单的神经系统检查。

**Patient:** Ok.

病人:好的。

*The results show that the patient is awake and* pupillary reflexes *as well as limb muscle strength are normal.*

检查结果显示:病人清醒,瞳孔反射及肢体肌力正常。

**Doctor:** Based on the results of the initial neurological examination, your conditions may be a hypertension-associated headache. We will give you oxygen and sublingual antihypertensive medication while we prepare to send you to the hospital for further examination and treatment.

医生:根据神经系统初步检查结果判断,您可能是高血压相关性头痛发作。我们先给予您吸氧和舌下含服降压药,同时准备送您去医院进行进一步检查和治疗。

🔍 **Key Words and Phrases**

**pupillary** ['pʊpɪlərɪ] adj. 瞳孔的

**reflex** ['riːˌfleks] n. 反应能力,反射作用

**associated** [əˈsəʊʃieɪtɪd] adj. 有关联的,联合的

**sublingual** [sʌbˈlɪŋgwəl] adj. 舌下的,舌下腺的

**Patient:** OK, please help me with the pain as soon as possible. I'm really under the weather.

病人：好的，请您尽快帮我止痛，我真的很难受。

**Doctor:** Painkillers cannot address the root cause of your illness. They will affect the professional's judgement instead. Sublingual antihypertensive medication will soon take effect. Please lie flat and have a rest. We have contacted the hospital for admitting and my colleague will do a CT scan of your head to check the secondary headache of hypertension.

医生：止痛药不能解除根本病因，反而会影响专业人员对疾病的判断，舌下含服降压药很快就会起效，请您平躺休息。我们已联系了医院准备接收，我的同事会对您进行头颅 CT 检查，排查高血压病引起的继发性头痛。

**Patient:** I see. Thank you!

病人：我明白了，谢谢医生。

## Useful Expressions

When did it occur? Have you had the similar experience

**🔍 Key Words and Phrases**

**under the weather** 身体情况很糟糕

**painkiller** ['peɪnˌkɪlə] n. 止痛药

**professional** [prə'feʃənl] n. 专业人士，内行；adj. 专业的，非业余的

**take effect** 生效，奏效

**contact** ['kɒntækt] v. 联系，联络；n. 联系，联络

**CT** (computed tomography 的简称) 计算机断层扫描

**scan** [skæn] n. 扫描检查，胎儿扫描检查

**secondary** ['sekəndri] adj. 继发的，次要的，辅助的

before?

什么时候开始出现症状的,您之前有过类似经历吗?

Do you have blackout, double vision or the feeling of objects spinning around you?

您有眼前发黑、重影或者物体旋转感吗?

Do you have chest tightness, chest pain or other symptoms?

您有胸闷、胸痛或其他症状吗?

Have you had any chronic diseases such as high blood pressure or diabetes?

您既往有高血压、糖尿病等慢性疾病吗?

Have you taken oral antihypertensive medication regularly? How has your blood pressure been?

您有定期口服降压药物吗,血压控制得如何?

Based on the results of the initial neurological examination, your condition may be a hypertension-associated headache.

根据神经系统初步检查结果判断,您可能是高血压相关性头痛发作。

## Section 8　Acute Chest Pain
## 急性胸痛

### Conversation

**Patient, female, 62 years old, suddenly had a sharp pain in her chest. Her family member called for emergency medical services.**

病人,女性,62 岁,突发胸部剧痛,家属拨打了 120 急救电话。

**Doctor:** Hello, I am a paramedic. What symptoms and feelings did you have?

医生:您好,我是急救医生。您有什么症状,感觉如何?

**Patient:** I suddenly felt sharp pain in my chest.

病人:我突然感到胸部特别痛。

**Doctor:** When did it occur?

医生:什么时候开始的?

**Patient:** About half an hour ago.

病人:大概半小时前。

**Doctor:** Which part of your chest was painful? Please point to the specific position.

医生:您胸部哪个地方有痛感,请用手示意具体部位。

**Patient:** Pain in the sternum, mainly behind the sternum, was very severe.

病人:胸骨处,主要是胸骨后面,疼痛非常剧烈。

**Doctor:** Can you describe the pain type? Is it dull, cutting, tearing or crushing pain?

医生:您能描述一下疼痛类型吗? 闷痛、刀割样痛、撕裂样痛,还是压榨样痛。

---

🔍 **Key Words and Phrases**

sternum ['stɜːnəm] n. 胸骨,胸片,胸板

tearing ['teərɪŋ] adj. 撕开的,痛苦的

crushing ['krʌʃɪŋ] adj. 压迫的,决定性的,支离破碎的

**Patient:** Pain in my chest like something was being pressed against it.

病人：像是有东西压得我胸口疼。

**Doctor:** Has the pain been continuous until now?

医生：疼痛一直持续到现在吗？

**Patient:** It is slightly relieved now.

病人：现在缓解一些了。

**Doctor:** How long did the crushing one last?

医生：这种压榨性胸痛大概持续了多长时间？

**Patient:** For about 20 minutes.

病人：大约 20 分钟。

**Doctor:** Did it radiate to the other part?

医生：疼痛是否向其他部位放射？

**Patient:** To the left arm.

病人：向左胳膊放射。

**Doctor:** Was the pain relieved by medication or on its own?

医生：胸痛是服药后缓解的还是自行减轻的？

**Patient:** I felt better when lying flat.

病人：我是平躺后感觉好一点儿了的。

**Doctor:** Did you have any other symptoms or discomfort besides chest pain?

医生：除了胸痛，您还有其他症状和不适吗？

**Patient:** I was nauseous, had a cold sweat, felt dying. My family said my face turned pale.

> **Key Words and Phrases**
>
> **slightly** ['slaɪtli] adv. 稍微，身材瘦小
>
> **radiate** ['reɪdieɪt] v. 辐射，发射，使向周围扩展

病人：当时我感到恶心、冒冷汗，有种要断气的感觉，家人说我的脸都变白了。

**Doctor:** Did you vomit?

医生：有呕吐吗？

**Patient:** No, I didn't.

病人：没有。

**Doctor:** Have you ever experienced chest pain?

医生：您之前有胸痛的经历吗？

**Patient:** I occasionally have dull pain that goes away with rest.

病人：我偶尔有点闷闷的痛感，休息一下就好了。

**Doctor:** What were you doing before the pain?

医生：您这次胸痛发作之前在做什么？

**Patient:** I was running.

病人：我在跑步。

**Doctor:** Have you had hypertension, diabetes or heart disease? Or any chronic or special medical conditions?

医生：您之前是否有高血压、糖尿病、心脏病史，或者慢性疾病、特殊疾病史？

**Patient:** I only have hypertension, no other diseases.

病人：我只有高血压，没有其他疾病。

**Doctor:** Do you take medication regularly?

医生：您有定期服药吗？

**Patient:** I don't take it every day, and I only take it when I have a dizziness.

病人：我不是每天吃，只有头晕发作时才吃。

**Doctor:** How old are you?

医生：您多少岁？

**Patient:** 62.

病人：62 岁。

**Doctor:** Got it. The nurse will measure your vital signs and I will perform a bedside electrocardiogram on you. Please cooperate.

医生：好的，护士现在为您测量生命体征，我为您进行床边心电图检查，请您配合我们。

**Patient:** OK.

病人：好的。

**Doctor:** Your heartbeat is fast, but your blood pressure is a little low. Based on your medical conditions, symptoms, physical examination and electrocardiogram indication, you may have suffered from acute myocardial infarction.

医生：您的心率快、血压有点低。根据您的病史、症状、体格检查及心电图结果判断，您可能是急性心肌梗死发作。

**Patient:** It's such a serious disease! Is it life-threatening?

病人：这么严重的疾病！我会有生命危险吗？

**Doctor:** Please try to remain calm. We will provide you with oxygen and intravenous medication. We will immediately send you to the hospital for further treatment with continuous electrocardiogram and vital signs monitoring. Please let me know if

---

🔍 **Key Words and Phrases**

**acute myocardial infarction** 急性心肌梗死

**electrocardiogram monitoring** ＜医＞心电图监测，心电监护

your chest pain <u>intensifies</u> or if you feel unwell on the way.

医生：请您尽量保持冷静。我们先给予您吸氧及静脉用药，为您进行持续心电监护和生命体征监测，并立即送您到医院进行进一步救治。途中，您如有胸痛加剧或者其他不适，请及时告知我。

**Patient:** OK.

病人：好的。

## Useful Expressions

Which part of your chest is painful? Please point to the specific position.

您胸部哪个地方有痛感？请用手示意具体部位。

Can you describe the pain type? Is it dull, cutting, tearing or crushing pain?

您能描述一下疼痛类型吗？闷痛、刀割样痛、撕裂样痛，还是压榨样痛。

Has the pain been continuous until now?

疼痛一直持续到现在吗？

Do you have any other symptoms or discomfort besides chest pain?

除了胸痛，您还有其他症状和不适吗？

Have you had hypertension, diabetes or heart disease? Or any chronic or special medical conditions?

您之前是否有高血压、糖尿病、心脏病史，或者慢性疾病、特殊疾病史？

**🔍 Key Words and Phrases**

**intensify** [in'tensifai] v. (使)加剧,(使)增强

Your heartbeat is fast, but your blood pressure is a little low. Based on your medical conditions, symptoms, physical examination and electrocardiogram indication, you may have suffered from acute myocardial infarction.

您的心率快、血压有点低。根据您的病史、症状、体格检查及心电图结果判断,您可能是急性心肌梗死发作。

# Section 9　Acute Abdominal Pain
# 急性腹痛

## Conversation

**Patient, female, 32 years old, had experienced dull pain in her abdomen 3 days ago. The pain suddenly intensified 20 minutes ago, so she called for emergency medical services.**

病人,女性,32 岁,3 天前腹部开始隐隐作痛,疼痛在 20 分钟前突然加重,因此她拨打了 120 急救电话。

**Doctor:** Hello, I'm Dr. Han. What seems to be the problem?

医生:您好,我是韩医生。您哪里不舒服吗?

**Patient:** I'm having serious abdominal pain.

病人:我腹痛得厉害。

**Doctor:** When did it occur?

医生:什么时候开始的?

**Patient:** Three days ago, my abdomen began to ache faintly, but the pain suddenly

> **🔍 Key Words and Phrases**
>
> **abdominal pain** 腹痛

worsened just now.

病人：3 天前我腹部开始隐隐作痛，刚才疼痛突然加重。

**Doctor:** Which part was painful? Please point to the position.

医生：腹部哪个位置痛？请指一下位置。

**Patient:** It wasn't fixed.

病人：位置不固定。

**Doctor:** Was your abdominal pain metastatic?

医生：是转移性的腹痛吗？

**Patient:** Yes. It was around belly button at the beginning and now it's in the lower right abdomen.

病人：是的，刚开始是肚脐周围痛，现在是右下腹痛。

**Doctor:** Is it stabbing, dull or colic?

医生：是刺痛、钝痛还是绞痛？

**Patient:** It is stabbing now.

病人：现在是刺痛。

**Doctor:** Got it. On a scale of 1 to 10, with 10 being the worst, what is the level of your pain?

医生：明白了。如果要给您的疼痛程度打分，1 到 10 分，10 分为最痛，您会打多少分？

**Patient:** It's about 8 now.

病人：现在大约 8 分。

**Doctor:** Did you have any other discomfort during the attack,

---

**🔍 Key Words and Phrases**

**metastatic** [ˌmetəˈstætɪk] adj. 转移性的，变态的，变形的，由转移所致的

**belly button** 肚脐

**colic** [ˈkɒlɪk] n. 绞痛，疝痛，疝气

such as nausea, vomiting or diarrhea?

**医生:** 发病过程中您有别的不舒服吗？比如恶心、呕吐或腹泻。

**Patient:** Yes. I started having nausea and diarrhea 3 days ago. I vomited several times when the abdominal pain was severe.

**病人:** 是的。3 天前我就开始恶心、拉肚子。腹痛严重时吐了几次。

**Doctor:** Have you had a fever, chills, or other discomfort recently?

**医生:** 您最近有发热、寒战或其他不适吗?

**Patient:** I have had a mild fever, poor appetite, but no chills.

**病人:** 有点低热,没胃口,不畏寒。

**Doctor:** What was your highest temperature?

**医生:** 您的最高体温是多少?

**Patient:** The highest temperature was 38 degrees.

**病人:** 我最高体温是 38℃。

**Doctor:** Have you seen the doctor or received treatment in the last 3 days?

**医生:** 您这 3 天来有就医和治疗吗?

**Patient:** No. I thought it was gastroenteritis, so I have taken anti-inflammatory medication by myself for the past 3 days.

---

🔍 **Key Words and Phrases**

**diarrhea** [ˌdaɪəˈrɪə] n. 腹泻;adj. 腹泻的

**chill** [tʃil] n. 寒冷;v.(使)变冷

**gastroenteritis** [ˌgæstrəʊˌentəˈraɪtɪs] n. 肠胃炎,胃肠炎

**anti-inflammatory** [ˌæntiɪnˈflæmətri] adj. 消炎的,抗炎的

病人:没有。我以为是胃肠炎,这 3 天里,我自己吃了消炎药。

**Doctor:** Have you had appendicitis, abdominal surgery or any other illness?

医生:您之前有阑尾炎、腹部手术史或其他疾病吗?

**Patient:** No, but I have had gallstone.

病人:没有,但我得过胆结石。

**Doctor:** OK, the nurse will measure your vital signs and I will palpate your abdomen. Please let me know if you feel pain.

医生:明白。护士会为您测量生命体征,我准备对您进行腹部触诊,疼痛时请告知我。

**Patient:** OK.

病人:好的。

*After the examination.*

*检查后。*

**Doctor:** Based on the results of physical examination and your symptoms, it is possible that your severe abdominal pain is related to appendix. However, there could be other causes, which I cannot rule out at the moment. We will give you fluids and some antidiarrheal, antiemetic and others to relieve your symptoms.

---

🔍 **Key Words and Phrases**

**appendicitis** [əˌpendəˈsaɪtɪs] n. 阑尾炎

**gallstone** [ˈɡɔːlstəʊn] n. 胆(结)石

**palpate** [pælˈpeɪt] v. 触诊

**appendix** [əˈpendɪks] n. 阑尾

**antidiarrheal** [ˌæntɪdəriːl] adj. <医> 止泻的;n. 止泻剂

**antiemetic** [æntɪmetɪk] adj. 止呕吐的;n. 止吐药

Please do not eat or drink anything until we get you to the emergency room.

**医生:** 根据体格检查结果和您的症状判断,您的剧烈腹痛有可能与阑尾相关,不过也不能排除其他病因。我们会为您输液,并使用止泻药、止吐药等药物以缓解症状。在我们送您到急诊室之前请不要进食或饮水。

**Patient:** OK, is it life-threatening?

**病人:** 好的,我会有生命危险吗?

**Doctor:** We will send you to the hospital as soon as possible, so <u>specialists</u> will do further examination to determine the cause of the disease and give you <u>appropriate</u> treatment.

**医生:** 我们会尽快把您送到医院,专科医生将为您做进一步检查来确定病因并给予适当的治疗。

**Patient:** Thanks.

**病人:** 谢谢。

## Useful Expressions

Which part of your abdomen is painful? Please point to the position.

您腹部哪个位置痛? 请用手指一下位置。

Was your abdominal pain metastatic?

您的腹痛是转移性的吗?

### Key Words and Phrases

**specialist** ['speʃəlɪst] n. 专科医生,专家
**appropriate** [ə'prəʊprieɪt] adj. 适当的,合适的

Is it stabbing, dull or colic?

是刺痛、钝痛还是绞痛？

On a scale of 1 to 10, with 10 being the worst, what is the level of your pain?

如果要给您的疼痛程度打分，1 到 10 分，10 分为最痛，您会打多少分？

Did you have any other discomfort during the attack, such as nausea, vomiting or diarrhea?

发病过程中您有别的不适吗？ 比如恶心、呕吐或腹泻。

Have you ever had appendicitis, abdominal surgery or any other diseases?

您之前有阑尾炎、腹部手术史或其他疾病吗？

I will palpate your abdomen. Please let me know if you feel pain.

我准备对您进行腹部触诊，疼痛时请告知我。

Based on the results of physical examination and your symptoms, it is possible that your severe abdominal pain is related to your appendix.

根据体格检查结果和您的症状判断，您的剧烈腹痛有可能与阑尾相关。

We will give you fluids and some antidiarrheal, antiemetic and other symptomatic medications.

我们会为您输液，并使用止泻药、止吐药及其他对症药。

Specialists will do further examination to determine the cause of the disease and give you appropriate treatment.

专科医生将做进一步检查来确定病因并给予适当的治疗。

# Section 10   Hematemesis
# 呕血

## Conversation

**Patient, male, 59 years old, suddenly had a stomachache, tightness in his chest and then vomited blood. His symptoms improved after hematemesis, but he couldn't move around properly. So, he called for emergency medical services.**

病人,男性,59 岁,半小时前突然胃痛、胸闷、呕血。呕血后,症状改善,但无法活动,因此他拨打了 120 急救电话。

**Doctor:** Hello, I'm Dr. Han. What seems to be the problem?

医生:您好,我是韩医生,请问发生了什么事?

**Patient:** Half an hour ago, I had stomachache and chest tightness, and then vomited blood. The symptoms improved after I vomited, but I couldn't move around properly because of dizziness.

病人:我半小时前突然感觉胃痛、憋闷,然后开始呕血。呕血后,我的症状改善了,但由于头晕,无法正常活动。

**Doctor:** Are you sure it was hematemesis instead of hemoptysis?

医生:您确定是呕血而不是咳血?

**Patient:** Yes, I'm sure because I saw the food I had eaten at lunch from the vomit.

> **Q Key Words and Phrases**
>
> **hematemesis** [ˌhiːməˈteməsis] n. 呕血
>
> **hemoptysis** [hɪˈmɒptəsis] n. 咯血,咳血

病人：是的，我确定，因为我从呕出的血液中看到了今天中午吃的食物。

**Doctor:** Can you estimate the approximate amount of blood you have vomited?

医生：您能估算一下呕血量大概是多少吗？

**Patient:** It was not very large and the color was rather bright.

病人：呕血量不是很大，颜色比较鲜艳。

**Doctor:** Were there any clots?

医生：有血块吗？

**Patient:** Some.

病人：有一些。

**Doctor:** Before vomiting, did you have any other symptoms, such as nausea, dizziness and weakness?

医生：请问您呕吐之前是否有恶心、头晕、乏力等其他症状？

**Patient:** I recently have had nausea, stomachache and dizziness.

病人：我最近感到恶心、胃痛和头晕。

**Doctor:** How has your bowel movement been these days?

医生：您这几天大便怎么样？

**Patient:** It has been dark and loose.

病人：比较黑，稀烂样。

**Doctor:** Have you ever had similar symptoms? Have you had

---

🔍 **Key Words and Phrases**

**approximate** [əˈprɒksɪmət] adj. 大约的，近似的
**bowel movement** 大便

stomach problem?

**医生**:请问您是否曾经有过类似的症状,有胃部疾病吗?

**Patient:** Yes, I have had <u>gastric ulcer</u> and bleeding before.

**病人**:是的,我曾经有过胃溃疡和胃出血的病史。

**Doctor:** Have you ever received any treatment or surgery?

**医生**:那您是否接受过治疗或者手术?

**Patient:** I have had medication treatment, but I have stopped it for a while.

**病人**:我曾经接受过药物治疗,但已经停药一段时间了。

**Doctor:** Based on your symptoms and medical history, our initial diagnosis is that you may have experienced <u>upper gastrointestinal bleeding (UGIB)</u>.

**医生**:根据您的症状和病史,我们初步诊断,您可能是上消化道出血。

**Patient:** I have vomited more blood than before, so I'm a little worried about my health.

**病人**:这次呕血比之前的量多,我有点担心我的健康。

**Doctor:** Don't be nervous. We will control your conditions with medications, and we will send you to the hospital for treatment as soon as possible.

**医生**:不要紧张,我们先用药物控制病情,同时会尽快送您到医院接受治疗。

---

### Key Words and Phrases

**gastric ulcer** 胃溃疡

**upper gastrointestinal bleeding (UGIB)** 上消化道出血

**Patient:** Do I need surgery?

病人：我是不是需要手术？

**Doctor:** It depends. Now we need to examine and treat you immediately to avoid serious complications.

医生：看情况。现在我们需要立即为您进行检查和治疗，避免出现严重的并发症。

## Useful Expressions

Are you sure it was hematemesis instead of hemoptysis?

您确定是呕血而不是咳血？

Can you estimate the approximate amount of blood you have vomited?

您能估算一下呕血量大概是多少吗？

Before vomiting, did you have any other symptoms, such as nausea, stomach pain, dizziness and weakness?

请问您呕吐之前是否有恶心、胃痛、头晕、乏力等其他症状？

Have you ever had similar symptoms? Have you had any stomach problem?

请问您是否曾经有过类似的症状，有胃部疾病吗？

Based on your symptoms and medical history, our initial diagnosis is that you may have experienced upper gastrointestinal bleeding.

根据您的症状和病史，我们初步诊断，您可能是上消化道出血。

# Section 11　Hemoptysis
# 咯血

## Conversation

Patient, male, 45 years old, suddenly coughed up blood which was bright red. He called for emergency medical services.

病人,男性,45 岁,突然咳血,血液为鲜红色,他拨打了 120 急救电话。

**Doctor:** Hello, what is the matter with you?

医生:您好,请问您有什么不适吗?

**Patient:** (*Shortness of breath*) I just coughed up a lot of blood all of a sudden.

病人:(*呼吸急促*)我刚才突然咳出了很多血。

**Doctor:** Just relax, please. We will take measures to help you. How much blood did you cough up?

医生:请您先放松,我们会采取措施来帮助您。您的咳血量有多少?

**Patient:** I don't know. I just coughed a few times and then I found a lot of blood.

病人:我不知道,我只是咳嗽了几声,然后就发现有很多血。

### 🔍 Key Words and Phrases

cough up 咳出或吐出

**Doctor:** Was there any <u>foam</u> or <u>sputum</u> in the blood?

医生：血里面有泡沫或者痰液吗？

**Patient:** Yes.

病人：有的。

**Doctor:** Have you recently experienced any discomfort, such as coughing, bringing up <u>phlegm</u>, chest pain or fever?

医生：请问您最近是否有咳嗽、咳痰、胸痛、发热等不适？

**Patient:** *(Shortness of breath)* Yes, I've been coughing and coughing up some sputum lately, but I haven't had chest pain or fever.

病人：*(呼吸急促)* 有，我最近一直有些咳嗽和咳痰，但是并没有胸痛、发热。

**Doctor:** Were there any other symptoms or discomfort before or after the hemoptysis?

医生：您咯血前后有伴随其他症状或不适吗？

**Patient:** I had a little <u>tickle</u> in my throat before it and I had a little shortness of breath and dizziness after it.

病人：咯血前喉咙有点痒，咯血后我觉得有点气促和头晕。

**Doctor:** Got it. Have you had any chronic diseases such as <u>tuberculosis</u> or <u>bronchiectasis</u>?

---

🔍 **Key Words and Phrases**

**foam** [fəʊm] n. 泡沫，泡沫材料，泡沫状物；v. 起泡沫，吐白沫

**sputum** [ˈspjuːtəm] n. 痰

**phlegm** [flem] n. 痰，镇定

**tickle** [ˈtɪkl] n. 搔痒，胳肢，愉快的情绪；v.（使）发痒

**tuberculosis** [tjuːˌbɜːkjuˈləʊsɪs] n. <医> 结核病，肺结核，痨，痨病

**bronchiectasis** [brɑŋkɪˈektəsɪs] n. 支气管扩张

医生：明白了，请问您是否有肺结核、支气管扩张等慢性疾病？

**Patient:** No, I haven't.

病人：没有，我没有得过这些病。

**Doctor:** Don't be nervous. I will treat you immediately. First of all, I need to measure your vital signs, <u>nasal</u> and <u>oral cavities</u>. I will also clean them if necessary. Then, I will give you some medications to stop the bleeding as well as give you oxygen.

医生：请您不要紧张，我会马上为您治疗。首先，我需要测量您的生命体征，检查您的鼻腔、口腔，必要时会对鼻腔、口腔进行清理。接着，我会给您使用一些止血药物，并给予吸氧。

**Patient:** I feel a bit short of breath.

病人：我感觉有点气促。

**Doctor:** Got it, I will give you an electrocardiogram. Please take deep breaths and relax.

医生：明白，我会为您做心电图检查，请您深呼吸并放松身体。

*After the simple first aid.*

*进行简单的急救处理后。*

**Doctor:** Do you feel any relief from the symptoms?

医生：您是否觉得症状有所缓解？

**Patient:** Yes.

病人：是的。

**Doctor:** Your condition has <u>stabilized</u> slightly. Next, we need to transfer you to a

> 🔍 **Key Words and Phrases**
>
> **nasal** [ˈneɪzl] adj. 鼻的，鼻音的
>
> **oral cavity** 口腔
>
> **stabilize** [ˈsteɪbəlaɪz] v. (使)稳定，(使)稳固

nearby hospital for further treatment.

医生：您的病情稍微稳定了。接下来，我们需要将您转运到附近的医院进行进一步治疗。

## Useful Expressions

Would you please tell me how much blood you have coughed up?

您能告诉我，您的咳血量是多少吗？

Was there any foam or sputum in the blood?

血里面有泡沫或者痰液吗？

Have you recently experienced any discomfort, such as coughing, phlegm, chest pain or fever?

请问您最近是否有咳嗽、咳痰、胸痛、发热等不适？

Were there any other symptoms or discomfort before or after you coughed up blood?

您咳血前后伴随有其他症状或不适吗？

Have you had any chronic diseases, such as tuberculosis or bronchiectasis?

请问您是否有过肺结核、支气管扩张等慢性疾病？

I need to measure your vital signs, nasal and oral cavities.

我需要测量您的生命体征，检查您的鼻腔、口腔。

I will give you some medications to stop the bleeding as well as give you oxygen.

我会给您使用一些止血药物，并给予吸氧。

## Section 12　Acute Airway Obstruction
## 急性呼吸道梗阻

## Conversation

Patient, male, 76 years old, had <u>dyspnea</u> 30 minutes ago, <u>accompanied</u> by violent coughing and <u>facial flushing</u>. He seemed to have phlegm <u>stuck</u> in his throat. His family member called for emergency medical services

病人,男性,76 岁,30 分钟前感觉呼吸困难,同时伴有剧烈咳嗽,面色潮红,似乎有痰卡在喉咙里,家属拨打了 120 急救电话。

**Doctor:** Hello, I'm the doctor in charge of this emergency care. What's the matter with him?

医生:您好,我是负责这次急救的医生。病人哪里不舒服?

**Patient's family member:** Hello, doctor. My grandfather has been coughing. He also had difficulty in breathing and seemed to have something stuck in his throat. We are very worried.

病人家属:您好,医生。我爷爷一直咳嗽,呼吸困难,感觉有

---

🔍 **Key Words and Phrases**

**airway obstruction** 呼吸道阻塞

**dyspnea** [dɪsˈpniːə] n. 呼吸困难

**accompany** [əˈkʌmpəni] v. 陪伴,陪同,伴随

**facial flushing** 面色潮红

**stuck** [stʌk] adj. 动不了的,被卡住的

东西卡在他喉咙里。我们很担心。

**Doctor:** When did these symptoms start?

医生：他是什么时候开始有这些症状的？

**Patient's family member:** About half an hour ago.

病人家属：大约半小时前。

**Doctor:** Did he have any other symptoms when he had difficulty in breathing?

医生：呼吸困难的时候，他还有别的症状吗？

**Patient's family member:** There was a slight <u>cyanosis</u> around his mouth.

病人家属：他嘴巴旁边有点发绀。

**Doctor:** Did he have any violent coughing, vomiting or choking?

医生：他有出现剧烈咳嗽、呕吐、呛水的情况吗？

**Patient's family member:** He has been coughing <u>violently</u> from then on, but no other symptoms.

病人家属：他一直剧烈咳嗽，没有其他症状。

**Doctor:** Did he take anything before the attack?

医生：发病前，他有吃什么东西吗？

**Patient's family member:** He took <u>antibiotic</u>.

病人家属：吃了抗生素。

**Doctor:** Why did he take this medication? What is its name?

---

🔍 **Key Words and Phrases**

**cyanosis** [ˌsaɪəˈnəʊsɪs] n. 发绀，苍白病，黄萎病

**violently** [ˈvaɪələntli] adv. 激烈地，暴力地，狂暴地

**antibiotic** [ˌæntibaɪˈɒtik] n. 抗生素，抗菌素；adj. 抗生素的

医生：他是因为什么服用这类药物，药物名称是什么？

**Patient's family member:** He has recently coughed up phlegm. So, he took this anti-inflammatory drug which seems to be cephalosporin.

病人家属：他最近几天咳嗽咳痰，所以吃了消炎药，好像是头孢类。

**Doctor:** Has he ever had any drug allergies?

医生：他既往有过药物过敏吗？

**Patient's family member:** I'm not sure.

病人家属：不是很清楚。

**Doctor:** I see. Has he had any respiratory diseases, such as asthma, bronchitis or emphysema?

医生：明白。他是否有哮喘、支气管炎、肺气肿等呼吸道疾病？

**Patient's family member:** Yes, he has had a recurrent cough.

病人家属：有的，他经常反复咳嗽。

**Doctor:** Can he speak now?

医生：他现在能讲话吗？

**Patient's family member:** Almost not.

---

🔍 **Key Words and Phrases**

**cephalosporin** [sefələʊˈspɔːrɪn] n. 头孢菌素

**respiratory** [rəˈspɪrətri] adj. 呼吸的

**asthma** [ˈæsmə] n. <医> 气喘，哮喘

**bronchitis** [brɒŋˈkaɪtɪs] n. 支气管炎

**emphysema** [ˌemfɪˈsiːmə] n. 气肿，肺气肿

**recurrent** [rɪˈkʌrənt] adj. 复发的，复现的，周期性的，经常发生的

**病人家属**: 几乎不能。

**Doctor:** Can he use body language?

医生: 他能用肢体语言表达吗?

**Patient's family member:** Yes, he can.

病人家属: 可以。

**Doctor:** I see. Let's examine him now.

医生: 我明白了,现在我们来给他做一些检查。

**Doctor:** Hello, do you have a tickle in your throat now?

医生: 您好,请问您现在感觉喉咙痒吗?

*Patient nods violently.*

*病人猛烈点头。*

**Doctor:** Which is more difficult for you, to <u>inhale</u> or to <u>exhale</u>?

医生: 您觉得吸气比较困难还是呼气?

*The patient inhales sharply several times and then coughs violently.*

*病人猛烈吸气几次,然后剧烈咳嗽。*

**Doctor:** I will look at your throat, listen to your lung and monitor your vital signs.

医生: 我将为您检查喉咙、听诊肺部,并监测您的生命体征。

*Patient nods again. After the examination.*

*病人再次点点头。 在检查之后。*

**Doctor:** His throat is red and

> **Key Words and Phrases**
>
> **inhale** [ɪnˈheɪl] v. 吸入,吸气
> **exhale** [eksˈheɪl] v. 呼气,放出,发散,发散出,放射,<医>渗出

swollen. He has thick phlegms and throat sounds, too. This may lead to his dyspnea. In addition, he has an obvious "three concave sign", rales in the lung and decreased breath sounds. His condition may be acute respiratory obstruction caused by red and swollen throat.

**医生**:他喉咙红肿,且有浓痰、喉鸣音,这可能跟他呼吸困难有关。另外,他有明显的"三凹征",肺有啰音,呼吸音减弱。他这种情况可能是喉咙红肿引起的急性呼吸道梗阻。

**Patient's family member:** What should we do?

**病人家属**:我们该怎么办?

**Doctor:** His heart rate is a little fast, and blood oxygen is a little low. We first try to suck out the phlegm, and then use medications to alleviate spasm, asthma and swollen throat to ease his dyspnea. At the same time, we need to send him to the hospital as soon as possible to do the relevant examination and further treatment. We will give him oxygen and monitor his vital signs throughout the process. If urgently needed, we will perform endotracheal intubation (EI) or tracheotomy to ensure that his

---

🔍 **Key Words and Phrases**

**swollen** ['swəʊlən] adj. 肿起的,涨满的

**concave** [kɒn'keɪv] adj. 凹的

**rale** ['rɑːl] n. <医>(肺的)水泡音,啰音

**suck out** 吸出,拔

**spasm** ['spæzəm] n. 痉挛,抽搐

**endotracheal intubation (EI)** 气管插管术

**tracheotomy** [ˌtræki'ɒtəmi] n. 气管切开术

airway is open. Please understand and don't worry. We will take all necessary first aid measures.

**医生**：目前他心率有点快，血氧有点低。我们先想办法帮他把痰吸出来，再用药解痉平喘、减轻咽喉水肿，缓解呼吸困难。同时，我们需要尽快送他去医院进行相关检查和进一步治疗。我们会全程给予吸氧和生命体征监测。如果情况紧急，我们将给予气管插管或气管切开以保证他的呼吸道通畅。请理解，不要担心！我们会采取一切必要的急救措施。

**Patient's family member:** I understand.

**病人家属**：明白。

*After a series of treatments, the patient has no cyanosis and his coughing has decreased.*

*经过一系列处理后，病人无发绀，咳嗽减少。*

**Doctor:** What's your feeling now? Can you talk?

**医生**：您现在感觉怎么样，可以说话了吗？

**Patient:** *(Nods and says weakly)* I feel better now.

**病人**：（*点点头，微弱地说*）感觉好些了。

**Doctor:** The patient's condition has been under control, but he needs further observation and treatment.

**医生**：病人的病情已得到控制，但需要进一步观察和治疗。

**Patient's family member:** Great, thank you! We will cooperate with the treatment.

**病人家属**：太好了，感谢医生，我们一定配合治疗。

---

**🔍 Key Words and Phrases**

**observation** [ˌɒbzəˈveɪʃn] n. 观察，监视

## Useful Expressions

When did the patient have dyspnea?

病人是什么时候开始呼吸困难的?

Did the patient have other symptoms while he / she was breathing difficultly?

病人呼吸困难的同时,伴随有别的症状吗?

Did the patient have any violent coughing, vomiting or choking?

病人有出现剧烈咳嗽、呕吐、呛水的情况吗?

Did the patient feel like something blocking his / her airway?

病人是不是觉得有东西堵住了他 / 她的呼吸道?

The patient has dyspnea, tachycardia, and cyanosis.

病人呼吸困难、心动过速及发绀。

We will monitor his / her vital signs throughout the process.

我们会全程监测他 / 她的生命体征。

Don't worry. We'll take all necessary emergency measures.

不要担心。我们会采取一切必要的急救措施。

The patient's condition has been under control now, but requires further observation and treatment.

病人的病情已得到控制,但需要进一步观察和治疗。

---

🔍 **Key Words and Phrases**

**block** [ˈblɒk] v. 堵塞

**tachycardia** [ˌtækɪˈkɑːdɪə] n. 心动过速

## Section 13    Airway Foreign Body
## 气道异物

## Conversation

**Patient, female, 50 years old, had dyspnea, felt like something was stuck in her throat. Her family member called for emergency medical services.**

病人,女性,50 岁,呼吸困难,感觉有东西卡在喉咙里,家属拨打了 120 急救电话。

**Doctor:** Hello, I'm a doctor at the <u>Emergency Center</u>. When did she experience dyspnea?

医生:您好,我是急救中心的医生。她是什么时候出现呼吸困难的?

**Patient's family member:** About half an hour ago.

病人家属:约半小时前。

**Doctor:** What was she doing before she had dyspnea?

医生:在出现症状之前,她在做什么?

**Patient's family member:** She was having dinner. Suddenly, she started coughing strongly, face turning red. After a while, she experienced dyspnea.

病人家属:她当时在吃晚饭,突然开始剧烈咳嗽,脸涨得通红,过一会儿就呼吸困难了。

**Doctor:** Has she had

> 🔍 **Key Words and Phrases**
>
> **Emergency Center** 急救中心

cardiovascular or lung diseases?

医生：她有心血管或者肺部疾病吗？

**Patient's family member:** No.

病人家属：没有。

**Doctor:** Has she ever experienced any foreign bodies in the airway?

医生：她之前有过气道有异物的经历吗？

**Patient's family member:** No, but she has had a poor appetite recently and may have accidentally swallowed something while she was eating.

病人家属：没有，但是她最近食欲不好，可能吃东西时不小心吞下异物了。

*Doctor turns to the patient.*

*医生转向病人。*

**Doctor:** Hello, I am a first aid doctor. Do you feel like a foreign object is stuck in your airway?

医生：您好，我是急救医生，您是否感觉有异物卡在气道里？

*The patient nods.*

*病人点点头。*

**Doctor:** We will perform some examinations and treatments on you. Please cooperate with us.

医生：我们需要对您进行检查和治疗。请您配合我们。

*The patient nods again.*

*病人再次点点头。*

**Doctor:** I will use this mouth

> **🔍 Key Words and Phrases**
>
> **appetite** [ˈæpɪtaɪt] n. 胃口，食欲
>
> **accidentally** [ˌæksɪˈdɛntəli] adv. 偶然地

opener to open your mouth and examine your throat and airway. Please avoid swallowing or moving. If I find any foreign object in your airway, I will try to remove it. Please follow my instructions to breathe and do not panic or struggle.

医生:我会用这个开口器来打开您的口腔,并检查您的喉咙和气道情况。请不要吞咽或做其他动作。如果发现您气道有异物,我会尝试将它取出。请您配合我的指令进行呼吸动作,不要害怕或挣扎。

*After examination, the doctor finds a piece of bone in the patient's airway and attempts to remove it with tools, but fails.*

*医生检查发现,病人气道里有一块小骨头,尝试用工具将其取出,但没成功。*

**Doctor:** I found a piece of bone in your airway, but I failed to remove it with the tools. Please remain calm, I will immediately try the Heimlich maneuver. Please cooperate with us.

医生:我发现您的气道中有一小块骨头,但我用工具取不出来。请您先保持冷静,我将立即采用海姆利希手法。请您配合我们。

*The patient nods again.*

*病人再次点点头。*

**Patient's family member:** What should I do?

🔍 **Key Words and Phrases**

**instruction** [ɪnˈstrʌkʃən] n. 指示,命令,操作指南,用法说明

**breathe** [briːð] v. 呼吸,呼气

**panic** [ˈpænɪk] n. 恐慌;v. 使惊慌失措

**Heimlich Maneuver** 海姆利希手法

**病人家属**：我需要做什么吗？

**Doctor:** You can help stabilize her body to prevent her from getting hurt. At the same time, you can comfort her and keep her calm.

**医生**：您可以帮忙稳定她的身体，以免她受伤。同时，您可以安慰她，让她保持镇静。

*After the doctor repeats the Heimlich Maneuver several times, the bone is successfully removed.*

*经过医生重复了几次海姆利希手法后，骨头被成功清除。*

**Doctor:** The foreign object has been cleared now. How is your feeling?

**医生**：现在异物已经被清除了，您感觉怎么样？

**Patient:** I'm feeling much better now, and I can breathe smoothly. But, I'm still a little dizzy and weak.

**病人**：我现在感觉好多了，呼吸顺畅了，但还是有点头晕、乏力。

**Doctor:** We will send you to the hospital for further examination and treatment. On the way, I will closely monitor your vital signs and your medical conditions.

**医生**：我们会尽快把您送到医院进行进一步检查和治疗。去医院的途中，我会密切观察您的生命体征和病情变化。

## Useful Expressions

I need to examine your breathing. Please try to remain calm and follow my instructions to breathe.

我需要检查您的呼吸情况。请您尽量保持平静，配合我的指令做呼吸动作。

I will use a mouth opener to open your mouth and examine your throat and airway. Please avoid swallowing or moving.

我会用一个开口器来打开您的口腔,并检查您的喉咙和气道情况。请避免吞咽或做其他动作。

If I find any foreign object in your airway, I will try removing it by tools.

如果发现您气道里有异物,我会尝试用工具将其取出。

If the foreign object cannot be removed by tools, I will immediately try the Heimlich Maneuver and other emergency measures. Please follow my instructions and try to relax.

如果异物无法用工具取出,我会立即采用海姆利希手法以及其他急救措施。请您配合我的指令,并尽量放松。

During the process, I will closely monitor your vital signs and your medical condition, and make corresponding adjustments and treatments as needed.

在急救过程中,我会密切观察您的生命体征和病情变化,并根据需要进行相应的调整和治疗。

## Section 14   Acute Exacerbation of Asthma
## 哮喘急性发作

## Conversation

**Patient, female, 36 years old, experienced chest tightness and dyspnea. Her family member called for emergency medical services.**

病人,女性,36 岁,感觉胸闷,呼吸困难,家属拨打了 120 急救电话。

**Doctor:** Hello! This is Dr. Han from the Emergency Center. What are your main symptoms right now?

医生:您好,我是急救中心的韩医生。请问您现在的主要症状是什么?

**Patient:** He … llo, doctor. I'm having difficulty breathing … and I've been wheezing …

病人:医生,您……好,我现在呼吸非常困难……一直在喘气……

**Doctor:** When did the dyspnea start?

医生:您是什么时候开始感觉呼吸困难的?

**Patient:** About … half an hour ago … I felt my chest tightening gradually … and then I started having dyspnea …

病人:大约……半个小时以前吧……我感觉胸部逐渐发紧……然后开始呼吸不畅……

**Doctor:** Do you have any other physical complaints or symptoms?

医生:您是否还有其他的身体不适或者症状?

**Patient:** I'm … feeling a little tired and a little dizzy.

病人:我……感到有些疲倦,还有点头晕。

**Doctor:** OK, do you have a cough?

医生:好的,请问您是否有

---

**Key Words and Phrases**

**wheeze** [wiːz] v. 喘息,发出呼哧呼哧的喘息声

**tighten** ['taɪtn] v. 收紧,(使)变紧,(使)绷紧

咳嗽?

*The patient has difficulty in speaking, so the family member answers instead.*

病人说话有困难,所以其家属代替回答。

**Patient's family member:** Yes, she has been coughing for some time.

病人家属:是的,她咳嗽已经有一段时间了。

**Doctor:** What medication has been used?

医生:她用过什么药物?

**Patient's family member:** She has been allergic, so she has taken oral anti-allergy medication.

病人家属:她一直过敏,所以口服抗过敏药。

**Doctor:** Has she ever had allergies or asthma? Has she ever had a similar attack?

医生:她是否有过敏史或者哮喘病史,是否曾经有过类似的发作经历?

**Patient's family member:** Yes, she has had an asthma attack once before, which was relieved by a rescue <u>inhaler</u>.

病人家属:是的,她之前也有过一次哮喘发作,经雾化吸入后缓解了。

**Doctor:** When was the last attack?

医生:她上次发作是什么时候?

**Patient's family member:** 2 months ago.

病人家属:2个月前。

**Doctor:** Got it. Does she have asthma medication with

🔍 **Key Words and Phrases**

**inhaler** [ɪnˈheɪlə(r)] n. 吸入器

her, such as an inhaler or emergency medication?

**医生**：明白。她是否随身携带了哮喘药物？比如吸入器或者紧急药物。

**Patient's family member:** No.

**病人家属**：没有。

**Doctor:** Has she recently been exposed to anything that might cause an allergy, such as pollen, pet dandruff or others?

**医生**：她最近是否有接触过导致过敏的物质？比如花粉、宠物皮屑或者其他物质。

**Patient's family member:** She has recently had a pet dog.

**病人家属**：她最近养了一只宠物狗。

*Doctor turns to the patient again.*

*医生再次转向病人。*

**Doctor:** OK, I'm going to measure your oxygen saturation, respiration, blood pressure and heart rate as well as listen to your lung.

**医生**：好的，我现在为您测量血氧饱和度、呼吸、血压和心率，同时进行肺部听诊。

*Patient nods. After the quick examination.*

*病人点点头。在快速检查之后。*

**Doctor:** Your oxygen saturation is a little low. Your breathing and heart rate are fast, and you have lots of rales, too. Based on your medical history, we use antispasmodic and asthma medications to

> **🔍 Key Words and Phrases**
>
> **pollen** ['pɒlən] n. 花粉，<虫>粉面
>
> **dandruff** ['dændrʌf] n. 头皮屑，头垢
>
> **antispasmodic** [æntɪspæz'mɒdɪk] n. 止痉挛的药

improve your breathing along with oxygen via mask.

医生：您的血氧饱和度有点低，呼吸和心率快，肺部听到大量的哮鸣音。结合您的病史，我们用解痉平喘类药物以及氧气面罩来帮助您舒缓呼吸。

*After a few minutes.*

几分钟后。

**Doctor:** Is there any improvement in your dyspnea?

医生：您的呼吸困难有改善吗？

**Patient:** Yes, it seems to be a little easier.

病人：嗯，好像轻松一点儿了。

**Doctor:** Great! Keep breathing slowly and deeply. We are going to take you to the hospital for further treatment. If your condition worsens, please let me know immediately.

医生：很好！保持缓慢深长的呼吸节奏。我们立刻送您到医院进行进一步治疗。如果情况恶化，请立即告诉我。

**Patient:** Thank you, doctor!

病人：谢谢您，医生！

## Useful Expressions

When did the attack start?

什么时候开始发作的？

Can you describe the symptoms in details?

您能详细描述一下症状吗？

Do you have dyspnea or wheezy now? How severe is it?

您现在感觉呼吸困难或喘息吗，严重程度如何？

Do you have chest tightness or pressure?

您有胸闷或胸部紧迫感吗？

Do you have any other symptoms, such as coughing or vomiting?

您有咳嗽或呕吐等其他症状吗？

Have you had dyspnea after inhaling irritants or allergens?

您是否在吸入刺激物或者变应原后出现呼吸困难？

Have you had any allergic reactions to your skin, such as rash or itching?

您的皮肤是否有红斑、瘙痒等过敏反应？

Do you experience persistent cough or shortness of breath even after asthma was relieved?

您是否在哮喘缓解后仍然有持续性咳嗽或者气短？

When was your last attack?

您上次发作是什么时候？

Based on your symptoms and medical history, you may experience an acute asthma attack.

根据您的症状和病史判断，您可能是哮喘急性发作。

## Key Words and Phrases

**irritant** ['ɪrɪtənt] n. 刺激物，刺激因素

**allergen** ['ælədʒən] n. 变应原

**rash** [ræʃ] n.（皮）疹，爆发

**itch** ['ɪtʃ] v. 发痒

**persistent** [pə'sɪstənt] adj. 持续的，坚持不懈的，持久的

# Section 15　Pneumothorax
# 气胸

## Conversation

**Patient, male, 65 years old, suddenly experienced shortness of breath and sharp pain in his upper left chest about an hour ago. The pain became more severe when he took deep breaths. His family member called for emergency medical services.**

病人,男性,65 岁,大约一小时前突然发生气促,左上胸有尖锐痛感,深呼吸时痛感加剧,家属拨打了 120 急救电话。

**Doctor:** Hello, I'm Dr. Han. I am told that you have dyspnea. Can you describe the symptoms for me?

医生:您好,我是韩医生。我得知您呼吸困难,可以描述一下您的症状吗?

**Patient:** Yes, doctor. I feels really hard to breathe, especially to take a full breath.

病人:好的,医生。我感到呼吸非常不畅,很难吸入一大口气。

**Doctor:** When did these symptoms start? Did they appear suddenly or get worse gradually?

医生:这些症状是什么时候开始出现的,是突然出现的还是逐渐加重的?

**Patient:** It started pretty

> **🔍 Key Words and Phrases**
>
> **pneumothorax** [ˌnjuːməˈθɔːræks]
> n. 气胸

suddenly about an hour ago. I just felt like I couldn't catch my breath.

**病人:**大约一小时前突然出现,我感觉喘不过气来。

**Doctor:** I see. Did you have chest pain or chest tightness? If so, where exactly was the pain located?

**医生:**我明白了。您是否感到胸痛或胸部发紧? 如果有,疼痛的具体位置在哪里?

**Patient:** I had a sharp pain in my left upper chest. It hurt me more when I tried to take deep breaths. I had a few coughs and chest tightness, too.

**病人:**我的左上胸有尖锐的痛感。当我试着深呼吸时,痛感会加剧,我还有些咳嗽和胸闷。

**Doctor:** What were you doing before the attack?

**医生:**您发病之前在干什么?

**Patient:** I was lifting heavy objects.

**病人:**我当时在提重物。

**Doctor:** How did you feel when you lay down after an attack?

**医生:**发病后,您平躺时感觉怎样?

**Patient:** I had more difficulty breathing when lying flat.

**病人:**平躺时呼吸更困难。

**Doctor:** Have you had any recent trauma or surgery to your chest?

**医生:**您的胸部近期是否受过伤或手术过?

**Patient:** No injuries or surgeries.

**病人:**没有受伤,也没有手术。

**Doctor:** Have you had any heart-related disease?

医生:您是否患有心脏方面的疾病?

**Patient:** No.

病人:没有。

**Doctor:** Have you smoked?

医生:您吸烟吗?

**Patient:** Yes.

病人:是的。

**Doctor:** How many years have you smoked?

医生:您吸烟多少年了?

**Patient:** About 20 years.

病人:大概 20 年了。

**Doctor:** Have you had lung disease like chronic obstructive pulmonary disease (COPD) or asthma?

医生:您是否有慢性阻塞性肺疾病、哮喘等肺部疾病?

**Patient:** Yes. I have had chronic obstructive pulmonary disease.

病人:是的,我有慢性阻塞性肺疾病。

**Doctor:** I see. Have you had a cough or coughed up blood?

医生:我明白了。您是否有咳嗽或咳血的情况?

**Patient:** I have had a cough, but I haven't coughed up blood.

病人:我有咳嗽,但没咳血。

**Doctor:** We need to give you an initial examination and

---

🔍 **Key Words and Phrases**

**chronic obstructive pulmonary disease (COPD)** < 医 > 慢性阻塞性肺疾病

monitoring.

医生：我们需要对您进行初步检查和监测。

**Patient:** OK.

病人：好的。

**Doctor:** You have weakened breath sounds on the left side of the lungs, and the breath sounds on the left upper lung seems to disappear. You have normal blood pressure and electrocardiogram, but increased respiration and heart rate, as well as low oxygen saturation. Your condition may be related to pneumothorax. We firstly give you oxygen to ease your dyspnea. At the same time, we immediately send you to the hospital for chest X-ray or CT and other further examinations to <u>confirm</u> the diagnosis and guide the precise treatment. So, you should continue to remain calm and cooperative. Don't worry. On the way, if necessary, we will take corresponding resuscitation measures.

医生：您的左侧肺部呼吸音减弱，尤其左上肺呼吸音消失；血压和心电图提示正常，但呼吸和心率增快，血氧饱和度较低。您的病情可能与肺部疾病有关。我们先给您吸氧以缓解呼吸困难，同时，马上送您到医院，进行胸部 X 射线或者 CT 检查，以及其他进一步检查，以明确诊断和指导精准治疗，您需要继续保持平静，配合我们。不要担心，路上必要时，我们会采取相应的抢救措施。

**Patient:** OK, doctor.

病人：好的，医生。

> **🔍 Key Words and Phrases**
>
> **confirm** [kənˈfɜːm] v. 证实，确认

## Useful Expressions

Do you feel any tightness or pain in your chest? If so, where is the pain located? How would you describe the nature and severity of the pain?

您感到胸闷或胸痛吗？如果有，痛处位于哪里，疼痛的性质和程度如何？

Have you had any heart-related disease?

您是否患有心脏方面的疾病？

Have you had any recent trauma or surgery to your chest?

您的胸部近期是否受过伤或手术过？

Do you feel pain or discomfort while breathing, especially in your chest or shoulder?

您是否在呼吸时感到疼痛或不适？特别是在胸部或肩膀。

Do you hear any sounds while breathing, such as wheezing or rough breathing?

您呼吸时是否会发出哮鸣声或粗糙的声音？

Have you had lung disease like chronic obstructive pulmonary disease or asthma?

您是否有慢性阻塞性肺疾病、哮喘等肺部疾病？

According to your conditions and examination results, if it is clear that you have suffered from pneumothorax, the doctor will carry out thoracentesis and other emergency resuscitation measures on you immediately.

如果根据您的情况和检查结果，能够明确您患有气胸，医

🔍 **Key Words and Phrases**

severity [sɪˈverəti] n. 严重

生会立即对您采取胸腔穿刺术等紧急抢救措施。

If you have tension pneumothorax and the compression area is relatively large, which poses threat to your health and life, the doctor need to perform thoracentesis on you to expel the excessive gas.

如果您是张力性气胸,压迫面积比较大,威胁到了您的生命健康,医生就需要为您进行胸腔穿刺术,将多余的气体排出。

# Section 16　Acute Respiratory Distress Syndrome
## 急性呼吸窘迫综合征

## Conversation

**Patient, male, 50 years old, was breathing faster with alarming tightness in his chest and blue lips. His family member called for emergency medical services.**

病人,男性,50岁,呼吸急促、强烈胸闷、口唇发绀,家属拨打了120急救电话。

**Doctor:** Hi, I'm an EMT. What's the matter with you?

医生:您好,我是急救医生,您哪里不舒服?

🔍 **Key Words and Phrases**

**acute respiratory distress syndrome** 急性呼吸窘迫综合征

**EMT** (emergency medical technician 的简称) 急诊医生

**Patient:** I am experiencing dyspnea with <u>intense</u> chest tightness and my heart is racing.

病人：我现在呼吸困难伴有强烈胸闷，心跳加快。

**Doctor:** When did these symptoms start?

医生：是什么时候开始出现这些症状的？

**Patient:** The symptoms started mildly yesterday and became worse half an hour ago.

病人：昨天开始出现轻微症状，半小时前加重。

**Doctor:** Have you had cardiovascular diseases or <u>pulmonary</u> infections?

医生：您患有心血管疾病或有过肺部感染吗？

**Patient:** I haven't had heart disease, but I have had acute <u>bronchopneumonia</u>.

病人：我没有心脏疾病，但有急性支气管肺炎。

**Doctor:** When did you have acute bronchopneumonia?

医生：您是什么时候患上急性支气管肺炎的？

**Patient:** Two days ago.

病人：两天前。

**Doctor:** Did you have any other symptoms?

医生：您还有其他症状吗？

---

🔍 **Key Words and Phrases**

**intense** [ɪnˈtens] adj. 强烈的，紧张的，激烈的

**pulmonary** [ˈpʌlmənəri] adj. 肺的，肺部的，有肺（肺状器官）的，患肺部疾病的

**bronchopneumonia** [brɒntʃˈɒpnjuːˈməʊnjə] n. 支气管肺炎

**Patient:** When I coughed up sputum and breathed, I needed to take deep breaths, which was hard for me.

病人：我咳痰和呼吸时，需要深呼吸，比较费力。

**Doctor:** Did you have breath-holding, chest tightness, irritability or fatigue?

医生：您有憋气、胸闷、烦躁不安或疲惫的感觉吗？

**Patient:** Yes.

病人：有。

**Doctor:** Let's monitor your vital signs and examine you.

医生：让我们来监测您的生命体征并做一些检查。

**Patient:** OK.

病人：好的。

**Doctor:** You are breathing rapidly, with retraction of supraclavicular fossa, substernal fossa and intercostal space. You also have very low oxygen saturation and a bit of cyanosis at the end of the extremities. You may have acute respiratory distress syndrome based on your medical history and the results of the preliminary examination. We first use oxygen therapy to correct the hypoxemia as well as some medications to fight the

---

🔍 **Key Words and Phrases**

**irritability** [ˌɪrɪtəˈbɪlətɪ] n. 易怒，过敏性，兴奋性

**supraclavicular fossa** <医> 锁骨上窝，锁骨上凹

**substernal** [səbˈstɜːnəl] adj. 胸骨下的

**intercostal** [ˌɪntəˈkɒstl] adj. 脉间的，肋间

**extremity** [ɪksˈtremɪtɪ] n. 手和足

**hypoxemia** [ˌhaɪpɒkˈsiːmɪə] n. 血氧不足，血氧过少

infection. Since your condition is critical, we need to send you to the hospital immediately for appropriate examination and further treatment.

医生：您的呼吸很快，锁骨上窝、胸骨下窝、肋间隙凹陷，血氧饱和度也很低，四肢末端有些发绀。根据您的病史和初步检查的结果判断，可能是急性呼吸窘迫综合征。我们首先用氧疗纠正低氧血症，并使用药物抗感染。同时，您的情况危急，我们需要第一时间送您去医院进行相应检查和进一步治疗。

**Patient:** Is my condition serious?

病人：医生，我的病情很严重吗？

**Doctor:** Try to relax. We are always by your side to monitor your vital signs. If necessary, mechanical ventilation will be used to supply you with oxygen.

医生：尽量放松，我们一直都在您身边，监测您的生命体征。必要时，我们会采用机械通气为您供氧。

## Useful Expressions

Do you have a rapid heart rate?

您是否心动过速？

Have you inhaled toxic gases or large amounts of smoke?

您是否吸入了有毒气体或者大量的烟雾？

Are you experiencing shortness of breath or chest tightness?

---

🔍 **Key Words and Phrases**

**mechanical ventilation** 机械通气

您是否有气短、气急以及胸闷？

Did you have breath-holding, chest tightness, irritability or fatigue?

您有憋气、胸闷、烦躁不安或疲惫的感觉吗？

Have you had cardiovascular diseases or pulmonary infections?

您是否有心血管疾病或者肺部感染？

Have you had trauma, burns or broken bones?

您是否有创伤、烧伤或者骨折？

Are your nails and lips blue?

您的指甲和口唇是否发绀？

You are breathing rapidly, with retraction of supraclavicular fossa, substernal fossa and intercostal space.

您的呼吸很快，锁骨上窝、胸骨下窝、肋间隙凹陷。

You may have acute respiratory distress syndrome based on your medical history and the results of the preliminary examination.

根据您的病史和初步检查的结果判断，可能是急性呼吸窘迫综合征。

If necessary, mechanical ventilation will be used to supply you with oxygen.

必要时，我们将采用机械通气为您供氧。

## Section 17   Acute Left Heart Failure
## 急性左心衰竭

### Conversation

**Patient, male, 65 years old, suddenly experienced dyspnea and chest tightness an hour ago. His family member called for emergency medical services.**

病人,男性,65 岁,1 小时前突然出现呼吸困难和胸闷症状,家属拨打了 120 急救电话。

**Doctor:** Hello, I'm Dr. Han from the Emergency Center. I was told that you are experiencing dyspnea.

医生:您好,我是急救中心的韩医生,我得知您呼吸困难。

**Patient:** Yes.

病人:是的。

**Doctor:** When did these symptoms start?

医生:是什么时候开始有这些症状的?

**Patient:** About an hour ago.

病人:大约 1 小时前。

**Doctor:** What were you doing an hour ago?

医生:1 小时前您在做什么?

**Patient:** Nothing in particular, I just lay down, resting.

🔍 **Key Words and Phrases**

**acute left heart failure** 急性左心衰竭

**病人:**没什么特别的,在躺着休息。

**Doctor:** What other discomforts did you have at the onset of illness?

**医生:**您发病时还有哪些不适?

**Patient:** I had chest tightness, dyspnea, and a feeling of suffocation, so I sat up. I breathed very fast and coughed up phlegm.

**病人:**我胸闷、呼吸困难,有种窒息感,所以我就坐起来,我呼吸很快,还咳嗽咳痰。

**Doctor:** What did the sputum look like? Did it have color?

**医生:**痰液是什么样的,有颜色吗?

**Patient:** Foamy, a bit pink.

**病人:**泡沫样,有些粉色。

**Doctor:** Did you have any symptoms a few days before the onset of the disease?

**医生:**发病前几天您有什么症状吗?

**Patient:** I've had a cold for the past few days and often had a dry cough as well as fatigue.

**病人:**我这几天感冒,常有干咳和乏力感。

**Doctor:** How has your urine output been recently?

**医生:**您最近尿量如何?

**Patient:** Less urine than usual.

**病人:**比以往的尿量少。

**Doctor:** Have you had edema in both lower extremities?

**医生:**您双下肢有水肿吗?

**Patient:** A little.

> **Key Words and Phrases**
>
> **suffocation** [ˌsʌfəˈkeɪʃn] n. 窒息
>
> **urine output** <医> 尿量
>
> **edema** [ɪˈdiːmə] n. <美> 水肿,浮肿,瘤腺体

病人:有点肿。

**Doctor:** Have you had a fever, <u>frequent micturition</u> or <u>urgent micturition</u> recently?

医生:您最近发热、尿频、尿急吗?

**Patient:** No.

病人:没有。

**Doctor:** Have you had hypertension or <u>coronary artery disease</u>?

医生:您是否有高血压或冠心病?

**Patient:** Both. I have had these diseases for ten years or so. I have often forgotten to take my cardiovascular medications recently because I have taken cold medicine.

病人:我两者都有,我有这些病已经十多年了。我最近在吃感冒药,经常忘记吃心血管方面的药。

**Doctor:** Have you ever had hyperthyroidism or lung disease?

医生:您有甲状腺功能亢进症或肺部疾病病史吗?

**Patient:** No.

病人:没有。

**Doctor:** We need to give you physical, electrocardiogram and other examinations.

医生:我们需要给您做体格检查、心电图检查等。

**Patient:** OK.

病人:可以。

**Doctor:** You have wet and cold skin, high blood pressure, rapid heart rate, a

> ### 🔍 **Key Words and Phrases**
>
> **frequent micturition** 尿频
> **urgent micturition** 尿急
> **coronary artery disease** 冠心病

lot of wet rhonchi in lung and low oxygen saturation. All these may be related to acute left heart failure. You should keep in a sitting or semi-sitting posture and take oxygen to increase the blood oxygen levels. At the same time, we will establish intravenous access and give you diuretics to help get rid of the excess water in your body. We will use vascular medications if necessary. Don't be nervous. We will escort you to the hospital as soon as possible for further examination and treatment.

**医生:**您皮肤湿冷,血压高、心率快,肺部有大量湿啰音,血氧饱和度偏低,考虑是急性左心衰竭。您应该保持坐位或者半坐位,我们先给您吸氧以提高血氧饱和度,同时为您开放静脉通道,并使用利尿剂,以帮助排出体内多余的水分,必要时我们还会给您使用血管治疗药物。不要紧张,我们会尽快护送您到医院,进行进一步检查和治疗。

**Patient:** Thank you, doctor.

**病人:**谢谢您,医生。

## Useful Expressions

Do you suddenly experience dyspnea or coughing?

您是否突然出现呼吸困难和咳嗽?

Have you had hypertension or coronary artery disease?

您是否有高血压或冠心病?

---

**Q Key Words and Phrases**

**diuretic** [ˌdaɪjuˈretɪk] n. <医> 利尿剂

**escort** [ˈeskɔːt, ɪˈskɔːt] v. 陪同,护送

What did the sputum look like? Did it have color?

痰液是什么样的,有颜色吗?

Are you experiencing rapid or irregular heartbeat?

您是否心跳过快且不规律?

How has your urine output been recently?

您最近尿量如何?

Have you experienced any signs of limb edema, ascites, or pulmonary rale?

您是否有下肢水肿、腹水或肺部啰音等体征?

Have you had discomforts, such as palpitations, chest tightness or chest pain?

您是否有心悸、胸闷、胸痛等不适?

Have you had edema in both lower extremities?

您的双下肢有水肿吗?

Have you had a fever, frequent micturition or urgent micturition recently?

您最近有发热、尿频、尿急吗?

Have you ever had hyperthyroidism or lung disease?

您有甲状腺功能亢进症和肺部疾病病史吗?

We will establish intravenous access and give you diuretics to help get rid of the excess water in your body. We will use vascular medications if necessary.

我们将为您开放静脉通道,并使用利尿剂,以帮助排出体内
多余的水分,必要时我们还会
给您使用血管治疗药物。

Ｑ **Key Words and Phrases**

ascites [æ'saɪts] n. 腹水

# Section 18　Shock
# 休克

## Conversation

Patient, male, 48 years old, has had a fever and headache for 3 days. He became <u>delirious</u> 2 hours ago and his family member called for emergency medical services.

病人,男性,48 岁,发热、头痛 3 天,神志不清 2 小时,家属拨打了 120 急救电话。

**Doctor:** Hello, what's wrong with him?

医生:您好,病人哪里不舒服?

**Patient's family member:** My husband lost consciousness just now.

病人家属:我丈夫刚才失去意识了。

**Nurse:** He has low blood pressure, fast breathing, weak and rapid pulse.

护士:他的血压很低,呼吸很快,脉搏微弱且快速。

**Doctor:** Based on his conditions, he has probably gone into shock. We will give him first aid treatment immediately by using medications to raise his blood pressure and restore his vital signs.

医生:根据病情,他很可能是休克了。我们需要对他进行抢救治疗,尽快用药物使他的血压上升、生命体征恢复。

> 🔍 **Key Words and Phrases**
>
> **delirious** [dɪˈlɪriəs] adj. 精神混乱的,非常激动的,极兴奋的,神不守舍的

**Patient's family member:** Please save him.

病人家属：请您救救他。

**Doctor:** Can you tell me something more about him before the attack?

医生：您能告诉我更多关于他发病之前的情况吗？

**Patient's family member:** My husband suddenly felt very weak, tight in his chest and had cold sweat, and then passed out.

病人家属：我丈夫突然感到非常虚弱、胸闷和冒冷汗，然后就昏迷了。

**Doctor:** Did the attack come suddenly or gradually?

医生：他的病是骤然发作还是缓慢发展的？

**Patient's family member:** He went into coma in a sudden.

病人家属：他是突然昏迷的。

**Doctor:** Did he feel faint or dizzy?

医生：他有没有感到眩晕或头晕？

**Patient's family member:** No.

病人家属：没有。

**Doctor:** Has he had any other diseases or other health problems before?

医生：他之前有什么疾病史或其他健康问题吗？

**Patient's family member:** He has coughed up sputum for this week, so doctor has given him penicillin.

病人家属：这个星期来，他一直咳痰。医生给他用了青霉素。

**Doctor:** Has he used penicillin today?

---

**Q  Key Words and Phrases**

**penicillin** [penɪˈsɪlɪn] n. 青霉素，盘尼西林

医生：他今天用了青霉素吗？

**Patient's family member:** Yes, he just came back from the injection in community clinic.

病人家属：是的，他刚才从社区诊所打针回来。

**Doctor:** Got it. Has he been allergic to drugs or plants?

医生：明白了。他是否有药物或者植物过敏史？

**Patient's family member:** No.

病人家属：没有。

**Doctor:** Has he been bleeding recently?

医生：他最近有出血症状吗？

**Patient's family member:** No.

病人家属：没有。

**Doctor:** Has the patient had heart conditions, such as palpitations, myocardial infarction or any other cardiac diseases?

医生：他之前有心悸、心肌梗死或其他心脏疾病吗？

**Patient's family member:** None.

病人家属：也没有。

**Doctor:** I see. Preliminary examination results show that his blood pressure drops sharply and he has low body temperature, swollen throat and bronchospasm. It is likely that he has gone into shock due to an allergic reaction.

医生：我明白了。初步检查结果显示，他血压骤降、体温

---

🔍 **Key Words and Phrases**

**preliminary** [prɪˈlɪmɪnəri] adj. 初步的，预备的

**bronchospasm** [ˈbrɒŋkəˌspæzəm] n. 支气管痉挛

低、喉咙水肿、支气管痉挛,可能是过敏引起的休克。

**Patient's family member:** What has he been allergic to?

病人家属:他是什么过敏?

**Doctor:** He may have been allergic to penicillin.

医生:他可能是青霉素过敏。

**Patient's family member:** It's not possible. He has used penicillin for these few days and he has been given a skin test every time.

病人家属:不大可能。因为他这几天都在用青霉素,而且每次都有进行皮试。

**Doctor:** The issue of human allergy to drugs is complex, which is beyond simple explanation.

医生:人体对药物的过敏问题很复杂,无法简单地解释。

**Patient's family member:** What should we do?

病人家属:我们该怎么办?

**Doctor:** We first help him lie flat to make sure his airway is open. Then, we will cover him with blankets to keep him warm. We've already given him medication to raise his blood pressure, and now we add anti-allergy treatment. All these emergency care will relieve his symptoms.

医生:我们先协助他平躺,保持呼吸道通畅,同时给他盖上毯子帮他保暖。我们刚才已经给他用了升血压的药,现在再对他进行抗过敏治疗。这些紧急措施能够缓解他的病情。

**Patient's family member:** Does he still need to go to the hospital for treatment?

病人家属:他还需要去医院接受治疗吗?

**Doctor:** Of course. We'll take him to the hospital as soon as possible, where the specialists will perform more examinations on him and address his problems. In the ambulance, we will monitor his vital signs, such as blood pressure, heart rate and breathing.

医生：当然需要。我们会尽快送他去医院，那里的专科医生会对他进行进一步检查以及对症治疗。在救护车上，我们会监测他的血压、心率和呼吸等生命体征。

**Patient's family member:** Thank you very much!

病人家属：非常感谢！

## Useful Expressions

Is the patient conscious or unconscious?

病人是否有意识？

Based on his conditions, he has probably gone into shock. We will give him first aid treatment immediately by using medications to raise his blood pressure and restore his vital signs.

根据病情判断，他很可能是休克了。我们需要对他进行抢救治疗，尽快用药物升高他的血压、恢复他的生命体征。

Has the patient had heart conditions, such as palpitations, myocardial infarction, or any other cardiac diseases?

病人之前有心悸、心肌梗死或其他心脏疾病吗？

Has the patient had lung infection or other infections recently?

病人最近有肺部感染或者其他感染吗？

Does the patient have symptoms, such as decreased blood pressure or cold limbs?

病人是否有血压下降和四肢冰冷等症状？

Did the attack come suddenly or gradually?

疾病是骤然发作还是逐渐发作的？

Has the patient had any recent injury, surgery or trauma?

病人最近有受伤、手术或其他部位的创伤吗？

Has the patient been allergic to drugs or plants?

病人是否有药物或者植物过敏史？

Preliminary examination results show that his blood pressure drops sharply and he has low body temperature, swollen throat and bronchospasm. It is likely that he has gone into shock due to an allergic reaction.

初步检查结果显示，他血压骤降、体温低、喉咙水肿、支气管痉挛，可能是过敏引起的休克。

# Section 19　Palpitation
## 心悸

## Conversation

**Patient, male, 55 years old, suddenly had an irregular racing heartbeat. So, he called for emergency medical services.**

病人，男性，55岁，突发不规律心跳加快，他拨打了120急救电话。

**Doctor:** I am a paramedic. Can you tell me how you are feeling?

医生：我是急救医生，您能告诉我您现在感觉怎么样吗？

**Patient:** My heart is beating rapidly and I think I'm going to faint.

病人：我心跳很快，我觉得我快要晕倒了。

**Doctor:** Can you describe in details what the rapid heartbeat feels like? Does your heart beat too fast or does it suddenly beat fast for a few times?

医生：您能详细描述一下心跳加速的感觉吗，是心脏一直跳得很快还是突然加速跳动几次？

**Patient:** It is paroxysmal rapid heartbeat.

病人：是一阵突然快速跳动。

**Doctor:** Is there a regular sudden increase in your heart rate?

医生：是有规律地突然心跳加速吗？

**Patient:** Not regularly.

病人：不规律。

**Doctor:** Have you recently experienced chest pain, shortness of breath, dizziness, nausea, vomiting and cold sweats?

医生：您最近是否有胸痛、呼吸困难、头晕、恶心、呕吐和冒冷汗？

**Patient:** I have been sweating a lot recently, and sometimes my breathing is a little fast. There are no other accompanying symptoms.

病人：我这阵子经常出汗，有时候呼吸有些快，没有其他伴随症状。

---

🔍 **Key Words and Phrases**

**paroxysmal** [ˌpærək'sɪzməl] adj. 爆发性的，阵发性的

**Doctor:** Have you had any diseases, such as high blood pressure, heart disease or hyperthyroidism?

医生：您有高血压、心脏病、甲状腺功能亢进症等疾病吗？

**Patient:** I have had hyperthyroidism.

病人：有过甲状腺功能亢进症。

**Doctor:** Have you taken any medications for it?

医生：您有服药治疗吗？

**Patient:** Yes, I have.

病人：有的。

**Doctor:** Have you had any changes in medication recently?

医生：您最近用药有没有变化？

**Patient:** I have stopped taking the medicine without consulting doctors for one year.

病人：我自行停药 1 年了。

**Doctor:** Have you had a <u>follow-up examination</u> to check on your <u>thyroid function</u>?

医生：后续有复查过甲状腺功能吗？

**Patient:** No.

病人：没有复查。

**Doctor:** Have you regularly had <u>caffeinated</u> <u>beverages</u> or

---

### 🔍 Key Words and Phrases

**follow-up examination** 复查

**thyroid function** 甲状腺功能

**caffeinated** [ˈkæfɪneɪtɪd] adj. 含咖啡因的

**beverage** [beˈvərɪdʒ] n. 饮料

alcohol?

医生：您是否经常摄入含咖啡因的饮料或酒精？

**Patient:** No.

病人：没有。

**Doctor:** Have you smoked?

医生：您是否吸烟？

**Patient:** No.

病人：我不吸烟。

**Doctor:** Have you had heavy stress in your daily work and life?

医生：您日常工作和生活压力大吗？

**Patient:** A little.

病人：有点。

**Doctor:** How did you sleep?

医生：您睡眠质量如何？

**Patient:** Often insomnia.

病人：经常失眠。

**Doctor:** Let's start by measuring your vital signs and doing an electrocardiogram to examine your heart activities.

医生：让我们先测量一下您的生命体征，并做心电图来检查您的心脏活动情况。

**Patient:** OK.

病人：可以。

---

🔍 **Key Words and Phrases**

**insomnia** [ɪnˈsɒmnɪə] n. <医>失眠，失眠症

**Nurse:** His blood pressure is normal, but his pulse is rapid and irregular.

护士：他的血压正常，但脉搏快且不规则。

**Doctor:** OK, the electrocardiogram also suggests that you have a tachycardia and have frequent <u>premature ventricular contractions</u> (PVCs). You may be experiencing an <u>arrhythmia</u>.

医生：好的，心电图也提示您有心动过速和频繁室性期前收缩，您可能是心律失常。

**Patient:** Why do I feel palpitations?

病人：我为什么会觉得心悸？

**Doctor:** Your palpitations may be caused by an arrhythmia, which means your heart's rhythm is abnormal.

医生：您的心悸可能是心律失常引起的，心律失常意味着您的心脏节律出现了异常。

**Patient:** What is the cause?

病人：这是什么原因呢？

**Doctor:** There are many causes for arrhythmia, including hyperthyroidism, chronic sleep deprivation, heavy stress or heart conditions. We need to take you to the hospital immediately for further examination and treatment.

医生：造成心律失常的原因有很多，包括甲状腺功能亢进、长期睡眠不足、压力过大或心脏方面的疾病。我们需要立即送

---

🔍 **Key Words and Phrases**

**premature ventricular contractions (PVCs)** 室性期前收缩
**arrhythmia** [əˈrɪθmɪə] n. 心律失常，心律不齐

您去医院进行进一步检查和治疗。

**Patient:** Do I need to do a lot of examinations?

病人：我需要检查很多项目吗？

**Doctor:** You may need to do some blood tests, such as thyroid function and electrolytes. You also need a cardiac ultrasound examination. Any of these abnormalities can cause palpitation.

医生：您可能需要做一些血液检查，比如甲状腺功能、电解质检查。同时，您还需要做心脏彩超。其中任何一项异常都可以引起心悸。

**Patient:** I see.

病人：我明白了。

**Doctor:** We firstly give you oxygen to make sure your oxygen saturation is stable.

医生：我们先给您吸氧以保证血氧饱和度稳定。

**Patient:** OK.

病人：好的。

**Doctor:** If there is any other discomfort on the way to hospital, please let me know at once. We will try our best to safely send you to the hospital for further examination and treatment.

医生：如果在去医院的路上出现其他不适，请立即告诉我，我们会尽力把您安全送去医院，进行进一步检查和治疗。

**Patient:** Thank you very much!

病人：非常感谢！

### 🔍 Key Words and Phrases

**electrolyte** [ɪˈlektrəˌlaɪt] n. <化> 电解液，电解质

# Useful Expressions

Can you describe in details what the rapid beating feels like?

您可以再详细描述一下心跳加速的感觉吗？

Does your heart beat fast or does it suddenly beat fast for a few times?

是觉得心脏一直跳得很快还是突然加速跳动几次？

Have you recently experienced chest pain, shortness of breathing, dizziness, nausea, vomiting, cold sweats, etc. ?

您最近是否有胸痛、呼吸困难、头晕、恶心、呕吐和冒冷汗等不适？

Have you had any diseases, such as high blood pressure, heart disease or hyperthyroidism?

您有高血压、心脏病、甲状腺功能亢进症等疾病吗？

Have you regularly had caffeinated beverages or alcohol?

您是否经常摄入含咖啡因的饮料或酒精？

Have you had heavy stress in your daily work and life?

您日常工作和生活压力大吗？

Let's start by measuring your vital signs and doing an electrocardiogram to examine your heart activities.

让我们先测量一下您生命体征，并做心电图来检查您的心脏活动情况。

The electrocardiogram also suggests that you have a tachycardia and have frequent premature ventricular contractions. You may be experiencing an arrhythmia.

心电图也提示您有心动过速和频繁室性期前收缩，您可能是心律失常。

There are many causes for arrhythmia, including hyperthyroidism, chronic sleep deprivation, heavy stress or heart conditions.

造成心律失常的原因有很多,包括甲状腺功能亢进、长期睡眠不足、压力过大或心脏方面的疾病。

We firstly give you oxygen to make sure your oxygen saturation is stable.

我们先给您吸氧以保证血氧饱和度稳定。

You may need to do some blood tests, such as thyroid function and electrolytes. You also need a cardiac ultrasound examination. Any of these abnormalities can cause palpitation.

您可能需要做一些血液检查,比如甲状腺功能、电解质等检查。同时,您还需要做心脏彩超。其中任何一项异常都可以引起心悸。

# Section 20    Vertigo
## 眩晕

## Conversation

**Patient, male, 73 years old, felt dizzy and nauseous after getting up in the morning. He walked unsteadily and had a tendency to fall down. So, his family member called for emergency medical services.**

病人,男性,73 岁,早上起床后感觉眩晕、恶心,走路不稳,有摔倒倾向,家属拨打了 120 急救电话。

**Doctor:** Hello, how can I help you?

医生：您好，请问您需要什么帮助？

**Patient:** I'm so dizzy that I can hardly stand steadily.

病人：我头晕得很厉害，快站不稳了。

**Doctor:** How long have you been like this?

医生：请问您这种情况持续了多长时间？

**Patient:** It started around 7 a. m. It is getting worse and worse.

病人：大约从早上7点就开始了，越来越严重。

**Doctor:** Was your vertigo accompanied by other symptoms such as headache, nausea or vomiting?

医生：您的眩晕是否伴随着其他症状？比如头痛、恶心、呕吐等。

**Patient:** Yes. After getting up, I have vomited once because of nausea. But I have had no headache.

病人：是的。我早上起床感觉恶心，吐了一次，但头不痛。

**Doctor:** Was your vertigo persistent or intermittent?

医生：您的眩晕是持续性的还是间歇性的？

**Patient:** Persistent.

病人：一直晕。

**Doctor:** Have you ever had hearing loss or tinnitus?

医生：您有没有感到听力下降或者耳鸣？

**Patient:** No.

病人：没有。

**Doctor:** What were your feelings when you had vertigo? Did you feel blurred vision or

> **🔍 Key Words and Phrases**
>
> **tinnitus** ['tɪnɪtəs] n. 耳鸣

spinning or unsteady?

**医生:** 您眩晕时有什么感觉,有没有感到视物模糊、天旋地转或者站立不稳?

**Patient:** No.

**病人:** 没有。

**Doctor:** Was your vertigo related to head movements or position changes?

**医生:** 您的眩晕是否和头部运动或体位变化有关?

**Patient:** It got worse when I turned around or got up.

**病人:** 当我转头或起床时会更严重。

**Doctor:** Did the vertigo come on suddenly or develop gradually?

**医生:** 这种感觉是突然出现的,还是慢慢发展的?

**Patient:** Gradually. I have ever had a vertigo once with mild symptoms.

**病人:** 慢慢发展的。我以前有过一次症状比较轻的眩晕。

**Doctor:** Have you received any diagnosis or treatment?

**医生:** 您有没有进行过诊断或者治疗?

**Patient:** I haven't been to hospital for that examination.

**病人:** 我没有特意去检查过。

**Doctor:** Do you usually keep the same posture for a long time, such as lowering head or working at a desk for a long time?

**医生:** 您是否经常长时间保持同一姿势? 比如长时间低头或长时间伏案工作。

**Patient:** Yes, often.

**病人:** 是的,经常这样。

**Doctor:** Have you ever had hypertension, diabetes, coronary artery disease, etc.?

医生:您是否有高血压、糖尿病或冠心病等?

**Patient:** No.

病人:没有。

**Doctor:** We will start by measuring your vital signs and neurological system.

医生:我们先给您测量生命体征,并进行神经系统检查。

**Patient:** OK.

病人:好的。

**Doctor:** Your vital signs are normal and the result of neurological test is negative. We will give you intramuscular drugs to relieve your dizziness and vomiting.

医生:您的生命体征都正常,神经系统检查结果是阴性。我们先为您肌内注射药物以缓解您的眩晕以及呕吐症状。

**Patient:** My problem can't be a cerebrovascular accident, right?

病人:我不会是脑血管意外吧?

**Doctor:** Don't be nervous. There are many causes for vertigo. For example, cervical spondylosis, Meniere's disease, vertebrobasilar artery insufficiency (VBI), etc. You should go to

---

**Q Key Words and Phrases**

intramuscular [ˌɪntrə'mʌskjələ(r)] adj. 肌内的

cervical spondylosis 颈椎病

Meniere's disease 梅尼埃病

vertebrobasilar artery insufficiency (VBI) 椎基底动脉供血不足

the hospital for further examination to determine the cause. For the time being, please continue to lie flat and try not to change the position of your body and head.

**医生：**别紧张。导致眩晕的原因很多，比如颈椎病、梅尼埃病、椎基底动脉供血不足等。您需要到医院进行进一步检查以明确病因，目前请您继续平躺，尽量不要改变体位和头部位置。

**Patient:** OK, I am feeling lighter now. Thank you, doctor.

**病人：**好的，我现在感觉轻松点儿了，谢谢医生。

## Useful Expressions

How long have you been like this?

您这种情况持续多长时间了？

Is your vertigo accompanied by other symptoms, such as headache, nausea or vomiting?

您的眩晕是否伴随着其他症状？比如头痛、恶心、呕吐。

Have you ever had hearing loss or tinnitus?

您有没有感到听力下降或者耳鸣？

What's your feelings when you have vertigo? Do you feel blurred vision or spinning or unsteady?

您眩晕时有什么感觉，有没有感到视物模糊、天旋地转或者站立不稳？

Is your vertigo related to head movement and position changes?

您的眩晕是否和头部运动、体位变化有关？

Do you usually keep the same posture for a long time, such as lowering head or working at a desk for a long time?

您平时有没有长时间保持同一姿势？比如长时间低头或长时间伏案工作。

Have you had hypertension, diabetes or coronary artery disease?

您是否有高血压、糖尿病或冠心病？

We will start by measuring your vital signs and neurological system.

我们先给您测量生命体征，并进行神经系统检查。

There are many causes for vertigo. For example, cervical spondylosis, Meniere's disease, vertebrobasilar artery insufficiency, etc.

导致眩晕的原因很多，比如颈椎病、梅尼埃病、椎基底动脉供血不足等。

We will give you an intramuscular injection to relieve your dizziness and vomiting.

我们先对您进行肌内注射以缓解您的眩晕及呕吐症状。

## Section 21　Sudden Cardiac Arrest
## 心搏骤停

## Conversation

**Patient, male, 79 years old, has had recurrent palpitations**

🔍 **Key Words and Phrases**

**sudden cardiac arrest** 心搏骤停

and chest pain in the past month. He suddenly lost consciousness and was unresponsive half an hour ago. His family member called for emergency medical services.

病人,男性,79 岁,最近一个月反复心悸和胸痛,半小时前突然意识丧失,呼之不应,家属拨打了 120 急救电话。

**Doctor:** The patient is unresponsive, not breathing and has no pulse. Let's perform cardiopulmonary resuscitation (CPR) and inject adrenaline.

医生:病人呼之不应,呼吸停止,动脉搏动消失。我们先为他进行心肺复苏,并注射肾上腺素。

**Nurse:** OK, right now.

护士:好的,马上。

*The patient's heartbeat and respiration restore after resuscitation therapy by the paramedics, but he has atrial fibrillation and hypotension.*

经医护人员抢救,病人恢复心跳和呼吸,但处于心房颤动和血压过低状态。

**Doctor:** Hello, please tell me something more about the onset of his illness.

---

**🔍 Key Words and Phrases**

**cardiopulmonary resuscitation (CPR)** 心肺复苏
**adrenaline** [əˈdrenəlɪn] n. <生化> 肾上腺素,<喻> 刺激物
**resuscitation therapy** <医> 复苏治疗
**paramedic** [pærəˈmedɪk] n. <美> 护理人员,医务辅助人员
**atrial fibrillation** 心房颤动
**hypotension** [ˌhaɪpəˈtenʃən] n. 血压过低

医生：您好，请告诉我您家人发病的情况。

**Patient's family member:** When my grandfather was chatting with me on the chair, he stopped talking all of a sudden, his face turning pale. He suddenly lost consciousness and did not respond even when we called him.

病人家属：当时我爷爷正坐在椅子上和我聊天，他突然一下子不说话了，脸色苍白，骤然丧失意识，我们叫他也没有反应。

**Doctor:** When did it happen?

医生：事情是什么时候发生的？

**Patient's family member:** Half an hour ago.

病人家属：半小时前。

**Doctor:** Did he have any discomfort before the attack?

医生：他发病之前有哪里不舒服吗？

**Patient's family member:** He has often complained about chest tightness and rapid heartbeats for the past month.

病人家属：他最近一个月经常说胸闷和心跳很快。

**Doctor:** Were the symptoms persistent or intermittent?

医生：这些症状是持续性的还是间歇性的？

**Patient's family member:** Intermittent.

病人家属：间歇性的。

**Doctor:** Has he had hypertension or heart problems?

医生：他是否有高血压或心脏方面的病史？

**Patient's family member:** He has had hypertension. Five years ago, he had a myocardial infarction.

病人家属：他一直有高血压，五年前曾有心肌梗死。

**Doctor:** Has he received the follow-up treatment?

医生：他有接受后续治疗吗？

**Patient's family member:** He only took medication when feeling sick in heart.

病人家属：他只有心脏不舒服时才吃药。

**Doctor:** Did you use first aid measures for his attack just now?

医生：刚才发病，你们有采取急救措施吗？

**Patient's family member:** We performed <u>external</u> chest <u>compressions</u> on him.

病人家属：我们对他进行了胸外心脏按压。

**Doctor:** He has atrial fibrillation and hypotension now. We will use <u>defibrillator</u> to deliver <u>electric shock</u> and inject medication to raise his blood pressure.

医生：他现在心房颤动、血压低。我们需要对他进行电除颤，同时给他注射药物以升高血压。

**Patient's family member:** OK.

病人家属：好的。

*After a while.*

过了一会儿。

**Doctor:** Your grandfather's blood pressure is gradually

---

🔍 **Key Words and Phrases**

**external** [ɪkˈstɜːnl] adj. 外面的，外部的；n. 外面，外部

**compression** [kəmˈpreʃn] n. 胸部按压

**defibrillator** [diːˈfɪbrɪleɪtə(r)] n.（电击）除颤器

**electric shock** 电击

rising now and sinus rhythm has been restored. We will send him to the hospital as soon as possible for further resuscitation and all kinds of examinations to find out the cause of his illness. His health can deteriorate at any time, and we will try our best to save his life.

医生：您爷爷的血压正在缓慢上升，心脏转为窦性心律了。我们需要第一时间送他去医院进行进一步抢救，做各类检查排查病因。但是他的病情随时都会恶化，我们会尽力抢救的。

**Patient's family member:** Thank you!

病人家属：谢谢您！

## Useful Expressions

The patient is unresponsive, not breathing and has no pulse.

病人呼之不应，呼吸停止，动脉搏动消失。

Let's perform cardiopulmonary resuscitation and inject adrenaline.

我们先为病人进行心肺复苏，注射肾上腺素。

When did it happen?

事情是什么时候发生的？

Did the patient have any discomfort before the attack?

病人发病之前有哪里不舒服吗？

Has the patient had hypertension or heart problems?

病人是否有高血压或心脏方面的病史？

The patient has atrial fibrillation and hypotension now.

> **🔍 Key Words and Phrases**
>
> **sinus rhythm** 窦性心律

病人现在心房颤动、血压低。

We will use defibrillator to deliver electric shock and inject medication to raise his blood pressure.

我们需要对病人进行电除颤，同时给他注射药物以升高血压。

# Unit 2

## Common Obstetric and Gynecological Emergencies
## 妇产科常见急症

### Section 1　Corpus Luteum Rupture
### 黄体破裂

## Conversation

Patient, female, 25 years old, suddenly experienced severe and <u>intolerable</u> abdominal pain an hour ago, feeling dizzy and nauseous, vomiting, and sweating heavily. She called for emergency medical services.

病人,女性,25 岁,1 小时前突发腹痛,剧烈难忍,伴头晕眼花、恶心、呕吐、大汗淋漓等症状,她拨打了 120 急救电话。

🔍 **Key Words and Phrases**

**obstetric** [əbˈstetrɪk] adj. 产科的
**gynecological** [gaməkəˈlɒdʒɪkəl] adj. 妇科的,妇产科医学的
**corpus luteum** 黄体
**rupture** [ˈrʌptʃə(r)] n. 断裂,< 医 > 疝气;v. 使破裂
**intolerable** [ɪnˈtɒlərəbl] adj. 不能忍受的,无法容忍的

**Doctor:** Hello, I'm paramedic. You called 120 about sudden abdominal pain and bleeding. Can you describe the position, symptoms and progress?

医生：您好，我是急救医生。您拨打 120 说突发腹痛和出血。您能描述一下疼痛部位、症状和发病经过吗？

**Patient:** OK, I felt a sudden and very severe pain in the lower part of my abdomen about an hour ago. The pain was so severe that I could hardly stand up. When I went to the bathroom, I found a small amount of vaginal bleeding.

病人：好的。大约一个小时前，我突然感到下腹部非常痛，痛得我几乎站不起来。当去洗手间时，我发现有少量阴道流血。

**Doctor:** Was the pain sharp or dull?

医生：是尖锐性痛还是闷痛？

**Patient:** Very sharp.

病人：很尖锐的痛感。

**Doctor:** Did the pain radiate to other parts?

医生：疼痛有放射到其他部位吗？

**Patient:** No, it didn't.

病人：没有。

**Doctor:** On a scale of 1 to 10, with the 10 being the worst, what was the level of your pain?

医生：1 到 10 分，10 分为最痛，您会给您的疼痛程度打多少分？

**Patient:** It was about 8.

病人：大约 8 分。

🔍 **Key Words and Phrases**

**vaginal bleeding** <医> 阴道出血

**Doctor:** Were there any other symptoms?

医生：有伴随其他症状吗？

**Patient:** I firstly had abdominal pain, feeling dizzy, having blurred vision, sweating heavily, and then had vaginal bleeding.

病人：开始是腹痛、头晕、眼花、大汗淋漓，然后出现阴道流血。

**Doctor:** Did you have a fever?

医生：有发热吗？

**Patient:** No.

病人：没有。

**Doctor:** Did you do strenuous exercise before the pain?

医生：您感到疼痛前有没有剧烈运动？

**Patient:** I did a high intensity of workout an hour ago.

病人：我 1 小时前做了高强度锻炼。

**Doctor:** Did you faint?

医生：当时您有感到头晕吗？

**Patient:** No.

病人：没有。

**Doctor:** What was the approximate amount of bleeding? Did you need to change sanitary protection frequently?

医生：出血量大约有多少，需要频繁更换卫生用品吗？

---

🔍 **Key Words and Phrases**

**strenuous exercise** 剧烈运动

**intensity** [ɪnˈtensəti] n. 强烈，(感情的)强烈程度，强度，烈度

**sanitary protection** 月经用品（卫生巾、卫生棉条等）

**Patient:** Not much, a pad was enough. But the bleeding is continuing.

病人：不多，我感觉用一张卫生巾就足够了。不过出血还在持续。

**Doctor:** Are you married?

医生：请问您结婚了吗？

**Patient:** Yes.

病人：是的。

**Doctor:** Do you have <u>sexual activities</u>?

医生：您是否有性生活？

**Patient:** Yes.

病人：有的。

**Doctor:** When was your last period? Are your <u>menstrual cycles</u> regular? Are you pregnant?

医生：您最后一次月经是什么时候，您的月经周期规律吗，有没有怀孕？

**Patient:** My periods are regular. The last one was about 2 weeks ago. I don't think I'm pregnant.

病人：我月经规律，最后一次月经大约是 2 周前。我应该没有怀孕。

**Doctor:** When did you have your last sexual activity?

医生：您最近一次性生活是什么时候？

---

### 🔍 Key Words and Phrases

**sexual activity** < 医 > 性活动

**menstrual cycle** 月经周期

**Patient:** Last night.

病人：昨晚。

**Doctor:** Have you ever been diagnosed with an <u>ovarian cyst</u> before?

医生：您之前被诊断过卵巢囊肿吗？

**Patient:** I haven't had it examined.

病人：我没有做过这方面的检查。

**Doctor:** Have you had any diseases or surgeries before?

医生：您之前有什么疾病或者手术史吗？

**Patient:** No.

病人：没有。

**Doctor:** Have you ever experienced pain like this before?

医生：您以前有过这样的疼痛经历吗？

**Patient:** No.

病人：没有。

**Doctor:** I am going to palpate your abdomen. Let me know if there's a particularly painful part.

医生：我准备为您进行腹部触诊，如果有特别疼痛的位置，请告诉我。

**Patient:** Ouch! It really hurts me when you press and release your hand on the lower right side of the abdomen.

病人：哎呀！您按压和松开右下腹时真的好痛。

**Doctor:** OK, the localized pain suggests that your pain may be in the right <u>adnexa</u>. And the

> **🔍 Key Words and Phrases**
>
> **ovarian cyst** 卵巢囊肿
> **adnexa** [æd'neksə] n.（器官的）附件

examination shows you may have <u>abdominal effusion</u>. I'm going to establish intravenous access and replenish fluids, and monitor your vital signs closely.

**医生：**好的，局部性疼痛表明您的疼痛可能发生在右侧附件区，而且检查结果显示您可能有腹水。我现在先为您开放静脉通道和补充液体，并密切监测您的生命体征。

**Patient:** OK, what disease do you think I have?

**病人：**好的。请问我得了什么病？

**Doctor:** Based on your medical conditions, symptoms and vital signs, you are likely to experience abdominal bleeding due to the rupture of the corpus luteum. In order to make a comprehensive diagnosis and prepare for surgical intervention, we need to perform some examinations on you, such as routine blood test, <u>blood coagulation</u>, <u>pregnancy test</u>, <u>pelvic ultrasound</u>, etc.

**医生：**根据您的病史、症状和生命体征判断，很有可能是黄体破裂导致的腹腔出血。但是，为了做出综合诊断，并为手术干预做好准备，我们需要进行一些检查，比如血常规检查、凝血功能检查、妊娠试验、盆腔超声等。

---

### 🔍 Key Words and Phrases

**abdominal effusion** 腹部积液，腹水

**blood coagulation** 血液凝固，血凝固，血凝结

**pregnancy test** 孕检，妊娠试验

**pelvic** [ˈpelvɪk] adj. 骨盆的，关于骨盆的

**ultrasound** [ˈʌltrəsaʊnd] n. 超声，超声波

## Useful Expressions

Is the pain sharp or dull?

是尖锐性痛还是闷痛？

Does the pain radiate to other parts?

疼痛有放射到其他部位吗？

On a scale of 1 to 10, with 10 being the worst, what is the level of your pain?

1 到 10 分，10 分为最痛，您会给您的疼痛程度打多少分？

Are there any other symptoms accompanying the pain?

疼痛有伴随其他症状吗？

Did you do strenuous exercise before the pain?

您感到疼痛前有没有剧烈运动？

What is the approximate amount of bleeding? Do you need to change sanitary protection frequently?

出血量大约有多少，需要频繁更换卫生用品吗？

Are you married?

请问您结婚了吗？

Do you have sexual activities?

您是否有性生活？

When was your last menstrual period?

您最后一次月经是什么时候？

Are your menstrual cycles regular?

您的月经周期规律吗？

Are you pregnant?

您有没有怀孕？

Have you ever been diagnosed with an ovarian cyst before?

您之前是否被诊断过卵巢囊肿?

I am going to palpate your abdomen. Let me know if there's a particularly painful part.

我准备为您进行腹部触诊,如果有特别疼痛的位置,请告诉我。

You are likely to experience abdominal bleeding due to the rupture of the corpus luteum.

您很有可能是因黄体破裂出现了腹腔出血。

# Section 2　Ectopic Pregnancy
## 异位妊娠

## Conversation

**Patient, female, 30 years old, experienced acute lower abdominal pain along with vaginal bleeding. She called for emergency medical services.**

病人,女性,30 岁,出现急性下腹痛及阴道流血,她拨打了120 急救电话。

**Doctor:** Hello, I'm doctor Han. What's the matter with you?

医生:您好,我是韩医生。您哪里不舒服?

**Patient:** I suddenly had lower abdominal pain along with

---

**🔍 Key Words and Phrases**

**ectopic pregnancy** 异位妊娠,子宫外孕

vaginal bleeding. I am worried that this may be something serious.

病人：我突然感到下腹部疼痛，同时还有阴道流血。我担心情况有些严重。

**Doctor:** When did these symptoms occur?

医生：您的这些症状大约是什么时候开始的？

**Patient:** About 30 minutes ago.

病人：大约30分钟前。

**Doctor:** Is it sharp or dull pain?

医生：是尖锐性痛还是钝痛？

**Patient:** Very sharp.

病人：很尖锐的痛。

**Doctor:** Please point to the exact part of the pain.

医生：请指一下疼痛的确切位置。

**Patient:** Here.

病人：这里。

**Doctor:** The pain on the lower left side is more pronounced, right?

医生：左下腹位置有比较明显的痛感，是吗？

**Patient:** Yes.

病人：是的。

**Doctor:** Do you have pain in other parts? Or has the pain shifted to another part?

医生：有没有别的地方也感到痛，或者疼痛有转移到别的位置吗？

**Patient:** The abdominal pain is relatively fixed.

病人：腹痛位置比较固定。

> 🔍 **Key Words and Phrases**
>
> **pronounced** [prə'naʊnst] adj.
> 明显的，显著的

**Doctor:** Is your pain accompanied by dizziness, blurred vision, urge to <u>defecate</u> or other discomfort?

医生：您腹痛时有伴随头晕、眼花、便意或者其他不舒服吗？

**Patient:** I have a little dizziness and a urge to defecate.

病人：我有一点儿头晕和便意。

**Doctor:** Which is less if comparing the amount of vaginal bleeding with that of <u>menstruation</u>?

医生：如果将阴道流血量跟您月经期的出血量比较，哪个血量少？

**Patient:** The vaginal bleeding seems to be less.

病人：这次阴道流血似乎比正常月经时量少。

**Doctor:** When was your last menstrual period? Have you missed it recently?

医生：您最后一次月经是什么时候，最近一次月经是不是没有来？

**Patient:** My last period was 5 weeks ago. I have missed this month's period.

病人：我最后一次月经是在5周前，这个月的没有来。

**Doctor:** Any nausea or vomiting?

医生：您有恶心、呕吐症状吗？

**Patient:** Occasional nausea, no vomiting.

病人：偶有恶心感，没有呕吐。

---

🔍 **Key Words and Phrases**

**defecate** [ˈdefəkeɪt] v. 排便，澄清

**menstruation** [ˌmenstruˈeɪʃn] n. 月经期间，月经，行经

**Doctor:** Have you had a <u>positive</u> pregnancy test or ultrasound examination?

医生：您有做过妊娠试验或者超声检查吗?

**Patient:** No.

病人：没有。

**Doctor:** Let's start with a pregnancy test.

医生：我们先做一次妊娠试验吧。

**Patient:** OK.

病人：好的。

**Doctor:** The result is positive, which suggests that you are pregnant. But there is no ultrasound examination to confirm whether the pregnancy is <u>intrauterine</u> or <u>extrauterine</u>. Have you ever had an ectopic pregnancy or <u>tubal</u> problems?

医生：妊娠试验结果显示阳性,提示您怀孕了,但还没有进行超声检查来确诊是宫内还是宫外妊娠。您之前有过异位妊娠或输卵管问题吗?

**Patient:** No.

病人：没有。

**Doctor:** I will examine your abdomen and <u>gynecology</u>. Can you cooperate?

---

🔍 **Key Words and Phrases**

**positive** [ˈpɒzətɪv] adj. 阳性的,积极乐观的,正面的,明确的

**intrauterine** [ˌɪntrəˈjuːtəraɪn] adj. 子宫内的

**extrauterine** [ˌekstrəˈjuːtərɪn] adj.(位于或发生在)子宫外的

**tubal** [ˈtjuːbl] adj. 输卵管的,管形的

**gynecology** [ˌɡaɪnɪˈkɒlədʒɪ] n. <医>妇科,妇科学

医生：我需要对您进行腹部及妇科检查，可以配合吗？

**Patient:** Yes.

病人：可以。

**Doctor:** Please tell me if you feel pain when I touch it.

医生：如果在我触碰时，您感觉到疼痛，请告诉我。

**Patient:** Got it.

病人：明白。

*The doctor starts examination.*

*医生开始检查。*

**Patient:** Ouch, my abdominal pain is obvious when you press on the left side.

病人：哎哟，您压左侧时，我腹痛很明显。

**Doctor:** Based on your symptoms of menopause, abdominal pain, vaginal bleeding and gynecological examination, you may have an ectopic pregnancy. This requires urgent medical intervention.

医生：根据您的停经、腹痛、阴道流血等症状及妇科检查结果判断，可能是异位妊娠，需要紧急医疗干预。

**Patient:** Oh my god. What should I do?

病人：天啊。我应该怎么办？

**Doctor:** For the time being, you should stay in bed and avoid strenuous activities, and we'll establish intravenous access and

---

🔍 **Key Words and Phrases**

**menopause** ['menəpɔːz] n. <医>停经，经绝（期），活动终止期，更年期，绝经期

**intervention** [ˌɪntə'venʃn] n. 介入，干涉，干预

replenish fluids. We will return to the hospital as soon as possible for further examination. Please let me know immediately if the pain gets more severe.

**医生：**目前您需要卧床休息，避免剧烈活动，我们将为您开放静脉通道及进行补液。我们要尽快返回医院进行进一步检查。如果疼痛加剧，请您立即告知我。

**Patient:** OK, thanks.

**病人：**好的，谢谢。

## Useful Expressions

When did these symptoms occur?

您的这些症状大约是什么时候开始的？

Is your pain accompanied by dizziness, blurred vision or urge to defecate, etc. ?

您腹痛时有伴随头晕、眼花、便意或者其他不舒服吗？

When was your last menstrual period?

您最后一次月经是什么时候？

Have you missed your period recently?

您最近一次月经是不是没有来？

Have you had a positive pregnancy test or ultrasound examination?

您有做过妊娠试验或者超声检查吗？

Based on your symptoms of menopause, abdominal pain, vaginal bleeding and gynecological examination, you may have an ectopic pregnancy.

根据您的停经、腹痛、阴道流血等症状及妇科检查结果判断, 您可能是异位妊娠。

This requires urgent medical intervention.

需要紧急医疗干预。

I will schedule an ultrasound examination for you to confirm the diagnosis.

我将会安排一次超声检查来确认诊断。

# Section 3　Abortion
# 流产

## Conversation

**Patient, female, 28 years old, was 12-week pregnant. She experienced lower abdominal pain and backache along with vaginal bleeding and white <u>tissue</u> discharge when waking up in the morning. She called for emergency medical services.**

病人, 女性, 28 岁, 怀孕 12 周, 早晨起床时, 下腹疼痛、腰痛, 伴有阴道流血和白色组织排出。她拨打了 120 急救电话。

**Doctor:** Hello, I'm an EMT. We've received a call from you regarding abdominal pain and vaginal bleeding. Can you tell me what has happened?

**医生:** 您好, 我是急救医生, 我们接到您关于腹痛和阴道流血的呼救电话。您能告诉我发生了什么事吗?

**Patient:** I am 12-week pregnant. I experienced very

> **Key Words and Phrases**
>
> **abortion** [ə'bɔː.ʃən] n. 流产
> **tissue** ['tɪʃuː] n. (动植物的) 组织, 薄纸, 面巾纸

severe lower abdominal cramps and backache when waking up this morning. When I went to the bathroom, I found heavy vaginal bleeding and some white tissues discharged.

**病人**：我怀孕 12 周。今早醒来时，我感觉到非常强烈的下腹绞痛和腰痛。当去洗手间时，我发现有大量阴道流血，而且排出了一些白色组织。

**Doctor:** How long has this been going on?

**医生**：这种情况持续了多长时间？

**Patient:** About 50 minutes.

**病人**：大约 50 分钟。

**Doctor:** Was this pain persistent or intermittent?

**医生**：疼痛是持续性的还是间歇性的？

**Patient:** It is paroxysmal, short-time intervals.

**病人**：一阵一阵的，时间间隔很短。

**Doctor:** If the bleeding is compared with your menstrual flow, which is more?

**医生**：如果将出血量跟您的月经量比较，哪个量多？

**Patient:** The bleeding was more than menstrual flow and there were many clots.

**病人**：这次出血量比月经量大，而且还有很多血块。

**Doctor:** Apart from the abdominal pain and bleeding, did you have any other discomfort?

> **🔍 Key Words and Phrases**
>
> **cramp** [kræmp] n.（腹部）绞痛，痛性痉挛
>
> **discharge** [dɪsˈtʃɑːdʒ] n. 排出物，获准离开，出院；v. 排出，允许……离开
>
> **interval** [ˈɪntəvl] n. 间隔时间
>
> **menstrual flow** 月经（流量）

医生：除了腹痛和流血，您还有其他不适吗？

**Patient:** I sweated heavily when I had abdominal pain. After the bleeding, I had some dizziness and vertigo.

病人：腹痛时我大汗淋漓，出血后有些头晕和眩晕感。

**Doctor:** Did you have any relief from abdominal pain or less bleeding after the discharge of the white tissue?

医生：您排出白色组织后腹痛有缓解或出血有减少吗？

**Patient:** I had some relief from the cramps, but I still have a vague pain in my abdomen. The bleeding is still as heavy as menstrual flow.

病人：绞痛有些缓解，但是我腹部仍有隐痛，出血仍如月经量。

**Doctor:** Are you sure you have seen the white tissue? What was its size?

医生：您确定看到了白色组织吗，它有多大？

**Patient:** Yes, I saw a white blister-like tissue.

病人：是的，我看到一个白色水泡样的组织。

**Doctor:** When was your last period?

医生：您上次月经是什么时候？

**Patient:** About 3 months ago.

病人：大约 3 个月前。

**Doctor:** What examinations have you had after pregnant?

医生：您怀孕后做过哪些检查？

**Patient:** I had an ultrasound and three early pregnancy tests at my 6 weeks'.

> **🔍 Key Words and Phrases**
>
> **blister-like** [ˈblɪstə(r)laɪk] adj. 水泡状

病人：我怀孕 6 周时，做了超声和早孕三项检查。

**Doctor:** What were the results?

医生：当时检查结果如何？

**Patient:** There was a little fluid in the <u>uterine cavity</u> and the <u>progesterone</u> was low.

病人：宫腔有点积液，孕酮偏低。

**Doctor:** Have you received treatment to prevent <u>miscarriage</u>?

医生：有进行安胎治疗吗？

**Patient:** Yes, I have been given intramuscular and oral medications.

病人：是的，我曾接受过肌内注射和口服药物治疗。

**Doctor:** What were the results of follow-up examination after the treatment?

医生：您接受治疗后复查情况如何？

**Patient:** I haven't been to the hospital for it this month.

病人：我这个月没有去医院复查。

**Doctor:** Got it. Let me examine you now.

医生：明白了，我现在给您检查一下。

**Patient:** OK.

病人：好的。

*After the examinations.*

*检查后。*

---

### 🔍 Key Words and Phrases

**uterine cavity** 子宫腔

**progesterone** [prə'dʒestərəʊn] n. 孕酮，孕激素，黄体酮，孕甾酮

**miscarriage** ['mɪskærɪdʒ] n. 流产，早产

**Doctor:** I can see blood clots and bleeding in your <u>cervical canal</u>. You may have had a miscarriage.

医生：我能在子宫颈管处看见血块和出血，您可能流产了。

**Patient:** Huh? What should I do?

病人：啊？我该怎么办？

**Doctor:** Firstly, I'd like you to lie flat to relieve your dizziness. Then, we are going to measure your vital signs and check if you have signs of going into shock. Next, we'll get you to the hospital as soon as possible to be treated by an <u>obstetrician and gynaecologist</u>. For the time being, we gain intravenous access and give you some fluids to ease your dizziness and potential blood loss.

医生：首先，我希望您能先平躺以缓解头晕。接着，我们要测量您的生命体征，并检查您是否有休克的迹象。然后，我们会尽快把您送去医院，交由妇产科专科医生治疗。同时，我们会为您开放静脉通道，给您输液以缓解头晕和潜在失血。

## Useful Expressions

Is this pain persistent or intermittent?

疼痛是持续性的还是间歇性的？

When was your last period?

您上次月经是什么时候？

---

🔍 **Key Words and Phrases**

**cervical canal** <医> 子宫颈管

**obstetrician and gynaecologist** 妇产科医生

Do you know you have been pregnant? What examinations have you had?

您知道自己怀孕了吗，做过哪些检查?

Have you received treatment to prevent miscarriage?

您接受过安胎治疗吗?

Are you sure you have seen the white tissue? What was its size?

您确定看到白色组织了吗，它有多大?

I can see blood clots and bleeding in your cervical canal. You may have had a miscarriage.

我能在子宫颈管处看见血块和出血，您可能流产了。

We are going to measure your vital signs and check if you have signs of going into shock.

我们要测量您的生命体征，并检查您是否有休克的迹象。

## Section 4　Precipitate Labor
## 急产

## Conversation

**Patient, female, 25 years old, has been pregnant for 36 weeks. She suddenly experienced abdominal pain with rupture of membranes. She called for emergency medical services.**

Q **Key Words and Phrases**

**precipitate labor** 急产，坠落产
**membrane** ['mem,breɪn] n.(动物或植物体内的)薄膜

病人,女性,25 岁,怀孕 36 周,突发腹痛伴胎膜破裂,她拨打了 120 急救电话。

**Doctor:** Ma'am, I'm doctor Han. Have you experienced any early signs of labor, such as contractions, water breaking and other symptoms?

医生:女士,您好! 我是韩医生。您是否已经出现了分娩的早期迹象? 例如宫缩、羊水排出等症状。

**Patient:** Yes, I have been pregnant and I feel fluid coming out and have abdominal pain.

病人:是的,我怀孕了,我感到有液体流出并且腹痛。

**Doctor:** When was your last menstrual period? When is the expected date of labor? How many weeks have you been pregnant?

医生:您的末次月经是什么时候,预产期是什么时候,现在是怀孕多少周?

**Patient:** My last period was more than 8 months ago. I have been pregnant for about 36 weeks.

病人:我最后一次月经是 8 个多月前,到现在怀孕大约 36 周了。

**Doctor:** When did you notice the water breaking and when did you start to have abdominal pain?

医生:您是什么时候发现有羊水流出,什么时候开始腹痛的?

**Patient:** I felt a bit wet about one hour ago. So, I packed my bags just yet to get ready to the

> **Key Words and Phrases**
>
> **bags just yet** 待产包,产前物品

hospital. I had abdominal pain about 25 minutes ago.

病人：大约 1 小时前，我感到有点湿润，就收拾待产包准备去医院。大约 25 分钟前，我感到腹痛。

**Doctor:** What color was the fluid? How often was your lower abdominal pain? Was it regular?

医生：羊水是什么颜色的，您下腹多久痛一次，有规律吗？

**Patient:** The fluid was clear at the beginning. The contractions came every 10 minutes, but more frequently now.

病人：羊水一开始是清的。每 10 分钟就会有一次宫缩，现在感觉更频繁些。

**Doctor:** Have you had any complications during your pregnancy, such as high blood pressure or diabetes? Have you ever received any special treatment or monitoring during this period?

医生：您孕期中是否出现过并发症？例如高血压、糖尿病等。在孕期中您接受过特殊的治疗或监测吗？

**Patient:** No.

病人：没有。

**Doctor:** Have you had <u>prenatal</u> examinations on time, such as ultrasound or <u>non-stress test (NST)</u>? Any abnormalities?

医生：您是否按时进行了产前检查？例如 B 超或无应激试验等。有异常吗？

**Patient:** Yes, I have had all the necessary examinations. My

---

🔍 **Key Words and Phrases**

**prenatal** [ˌpriːˈneɪtl] adj. 出生前的，胎儿期的
**non-stress test (NST)** 无应激试验，常被用于过期妊娠时对胎儿健康状况的评估

pregnancy went well.

**病人:** 是的, 我做了所有必要的检查。孕期都很顺利。

**Doctor:** Do you have a birth plan or any special requirements for delivery?

**医生:** 您有分娩计划或特殊要求吗?

**Patient:** I hope to have a full-term natural labor.

**病人:** 我希望能足月顺产。

**Doctor:** OK, the nurse is going to measure your vital signs. Let me examine your abdomen and fetal heart rate.

**医生:** 好的, 护士要测量一下您的生命体征。让我来检查一下您的腹部和胎心率。

**Patient:** OK.

**病人:** 好的。

**Doctor:** Your pulse is a little fast, and your blood pressure is slightly high. The contractions are very regular. The fetal heart rate is normal.

**医生:** 您的脉搏有些快, 血压也略高, 宫缩非常规律, 胎心率正常。

**Patient:** Will I have pre-term labor? If possible, please take measures to help me.

**病人:** 我是否会早产? 如果可以的话, 请您采取措施帮帮我。

---

🔍 **Key Words and Phrases**

**full-term** [ful tə:m] adj.(怀孕)足月的
**natural labor** 顺产
**fetal heart rate** <妇产> 胎心率

**Doctor:** Try to relax. I'm going to give you some intramuscular and intravenous medications to accelerate fetal lung maturation and inhibit contractions. We will transport you to the hospital for further treatment as soon as possible.

**医生：**尽量放松。我会为您肌内注射和静脉注射药物以促进胎肺成熟和抑制宫缩。我们会尽快把您送去医院接受进一步治疗。

**Patient:** Will my baby be all right? I'm very worried.

**病人：**我的孩子会没事吗？我很担心。

**Doctor:** I understand. For the sake of the baby, please try to stay calm. We will monitor the fetal heart rate and contractions closely.

**医生：**我知道您一定很害怕，但是为了孩子，请您尽量保持冷静。我们会密切监测胎心率和宫缩情况。

*On the way to the hospital.*

*去医院的途中。*

**Patient:** I feel the abdominal pain is more serious.

**病人：**我感觉腹痛加重了。

**Doctor:** Please remain calm. You seem to be in active labor and it is progressing very rapidly. We call this precipitate labor. I will check the dilatation of your cervix.

---

🔍 **Key Words and Phrases**

**maturation** [ˌmætʃuˈreɪʃn] n. 成熟，化脓

**inhibit** [ɪnˈhɪbɪt] v. 抑制，禁止

**dilatation** [ˌdaɪləˈteɪʃn] n.（中空器官或空洞）扩张，膨胀，扩张过程

**cervix** [ˈsɜːvɪks] n. 子宫颈，颈部

医生：请保持冷静。您似乎正在进入分娩活跃阶段，并且进展非常迅速，我们称此为急产。我将检查您宫颈的扩张程度。

**Patient:** Oh, my God. My abdominal pain is severe and my urge to push is too strong. Please help me!

病人：天呐！我腹痛严重，而且很想用力！请帮帮我！

**Doctor:** Your uterus is fully dilated and the baby's head is there. Your baby is going to be born immediately. We will prepare for an emergency delivery. Before we get ready for your labor, please try not to push too hard.

医生：您的子宫已经全面扩张，能看到胎头了。新生儿马上要出生了，我们需要准备应急分娩。在我们做好接生准备之前，您尽量不要用力。

**Patient:** I can't stop pushing.

病人：我无法停止用力！

**Doctor:** Stay calm and try to breathe deeply. We'll take care of you and your baby. When the next contraction comes, please hold your breath and push. We'll guide you to deliver as gently as possible.

医生：请保持冷静，尽量深呼吸。我们会照顾好您和您的孩子。当下一次宫缩来时，请您屏气用力。我们会引导您尽可能温和地分娩。

**Patient:** OK.

病人：好的。

**Doctor:** Great! Here comes the contraction, and please hold your breath and push.

> **Key Words and Phrases**
>
> **uterus** [ˈjuːtərəs] n. <解> 子宫
> **dilate** [daɪˈleɪt] v. 使扩大，使膨胀，扩张

医生：很好! 宫缩来了,请屏住呼吸,用力。

*Patient holds breath and pushes.*

病人屏气用力。

**Doctor:** Well done! Your baby is born. You have given birth a healthy baby girl. Congratulations! I'm going to cut the umbilical cord and we're going to clean the baby's airway and keep her warm. How do you feel?

医生：您做得很好! 您的孩子出生了。恭喜您生了一个健康的女孩! 现在我将剪断脐带,我们会为新生儿清理呼吸道并保暖。您感觉怎么样?

**Patient:** I feel a little dizzy, but I'm glad the delivery went smoothly. How is my baby?

病人：我感到有点头晕,但也很开心这一切都很顺利。我的孩子还好吗?

**Doctor:** She seems fine. We will help you to expel the placenta.

医生：她看起来很好,我们将协助您排出胎盘。

**Patient:** Thank you, I feel better now.

病人：谢谢您,我现在感觉好一点儿了。

## Useful Expressions

Have you experienced any early signs of labor, such as contractions, water breaking out or other symptoms?

您是否已经出现了分娩的早期迹象? 例如宫

> 🔍 **Key Words and Phrases**
>
> **umbilical cord** 脐带
> **placenta** [plə'sentə] n. 胎盘,胎座

缩、羊水排出等症状。

When was your last menstrual period?

您的末次月经是什么时候？

When is the expected date of labor?

您的预产期是什么时候？

How many weeks have you been pregnant?

您现在是怀孕多少周？

What color is the amniotic fluid?

羊水是什么颜色的？

Is your abdominal pain regular?

您腹痛有规律吗？

How often do you have lower abdominal pain?

您下腹多久痛一次？

Have you had any complications during your pregnancy, such as high blood pressure or diabetes?

您孕期是否出现过高血压、糖尿病等并发症？

Have you ever received treatment or monitoring during your pregnancy?

您在孕期中接受过治疗或监测吗？

Have you had your prenatal examinations on time, such as ultrasound or non-stress test? Any abnormalities?

您是否按时进行了产前检查？例如 B 超或无应激试验等。有异常吗？

Do you have a birth plan or any special requirements for delivery?

您有分娩计划或特殊要求吗？

Let me examine your abdomen and fetal heart rate.

让我来检查一下您的腹部和胎心率。

The contractions are very regular, and your fetal heart rate is normal.

您宫缩非常规律,胎心率正常。

I'm going to give you some intramuscular and intravenous medications to accelerate fetal lung maturation and inhibit contractions.

我会为您肌内注射和静脉注射药物以促进胎肺成熟和抑制宫缩。

You seem to be in active labor and it is progressing very rapidly. We call this precipitate labor. I will examine the dilatation of your cervix.

您似乎正在进入分娩活跃阶段,并且进展非常迅速,我们称此为急产。我将检查您宫颈的扩张程度。

Don't worry! I will guide you through the labor process.

别担心! 我会引导您完成分娩过程。

When the next contraction comes, please hold your breath and push.

当下一次宫缩来时,请您屏气用力。

# Unit 3

## Common Pediatric Emergencies
## 儿科常见急症

### Section 1　Asphyxia of Newborn
### 新生儿窒息

#### Conversation

Patient, female, a <u>newborn</u> baby, was born at home, and was experiencing difficulty breathing. Her family member called for emergency medical services

患儿，女性，新生儿，在家中出生，出现呼吸困难的症状，家属拨打了120急救电话。

**Doctor:** Hello, I'm Li Hua, a paramedic. We received a call about a newborn possibly having difficulty breathing. Can you tell

---

🔍 **Key Words and Phrases**

**pediatric** [ˌpiːdɪˈætrɪk] adj. 小儿科的
**asphyxia** [æsˈfɪksɪə] n. <医> 窒息，血液中缺氧，无脉
**newborn** [ˈnjuːbɔːn] n. 婴儿

me what happened?

**医生:** 您好! 我叫李华, 是一名急救医生。我们接到电话说有新生儿疑似呼吸困难, 您能告诉我发生了什么事吗?

**Patient's family member:** Yes, our baby girl was just born, but she's not crying or breathing well. She's gasping and her lips and fingertips are blue. We're really worried.

**病人家属:** 我们的孩子刚刚出生, 但是她没有哭, 呼吸也不顺畅, 喘不上气来, 嘴唇和指尖也有点发青。我们非常担心。

**Doctor:** I understand your concern. Let's work together to help your baby. Now I'll perform a quick assessment of the newborn's responsiveness, breathing, and color. And my colleague is going to administer oxygen to her and gently stimulate her to breathe.

**医生:** 我理解您的担心。让我们一起来帮助您的孩子。我现在要进行新生儿反应、呼吸和颜色的快速评估。我的同事会为她提供氧气, 并轻柔地刺激她开始呼吸。

*The nurse starts providing necessary cares, such as clearing the baby's airway, providing stimulation like tapping the feet, and giving oxygen.*

*护士开始进行必要的护理, 比如清理新生儿的呼吸道, 通过拍打足底等方式刺激呼吸, 供给氧气。*

**Doctor:** The good news is she's responding to the oxygen. I'm detecting a heartbeat and she's trying to breathe now. Can you please tell me if the baby

> **🔍 Key Words and Phrases**
>
> **gasp** [gɑ:sp] v. (因惊讶或疼痛) 喘气
>
> **assessment** [əˈsesmənt] n. 评估
>
> **responsiveness** [rɪˈspɒnsɪvnəs] n. 反应
>
> **stimulate** [ˈstɪmjuleɪt] v. 刺激

was born full-term or premature?

医生:好消息是她对给氧有反应。我能检测到她的心跳,她也在努力试着呼吸了。您能告诉我新生儿是足月出生还是早产吗?

**Patient's family member:** She was born full-term, just a few days past her due date.

病人家属:她是足月出生,已经过了预产期几天了。

**Doctor:** Got it. Were there any special conditions when she was born?

医生:好的,了解。她出生的时候有没有什么异常的情况?

**Patient's family member:** The umbilical cord was wrapped around her neck twice.

病人家属:当时脐带绕颈两周。

**Doctor:** Did her mother have any diseases before delivery, such as gestational diabetes, or anemia?

医生:产妇生产前有没有一些全身性疾病?比如妊娠糖尿病或贫血。

**Patient's family member:** No, everything is fine.

病人家属:没有,一切正常。

**Doctor:** OK, got it. We're going to transport her to the hospital right away for further treatment. She appears stable but still at risk due to suspected asphyxia at birth.

医生:好的,了解。我们现在要尽快将她转送到医院进行进一步治疗。她现

> 🔍 **Key Words and Phrases**
>
> **gestational** [dʒeˈsteɪʃənəl] adj. 妊娠期的
>
> **diabetes** [ˌdaɪəˈbiːtiːz] n. 糖尿病
>
> **anemia** [əˈniːmiːə] n. 贫血症

在情况稳定,但由于出生时疑似出现窒息,所以还存在一定的风险。

**Patient's family member:** We were so scared. Will she be fine?

**病人家属**:我们当时吓坏了。她会没事的吧?

**Doctor:** The doctors will do a full examination at the hospital. I know it's hard, but try to stay calm for her.

**医生**:医生会在医院给她进行全面检查的。我知道这很难,但还是请你们尽量保持冷静。

**Patient's family member:** Thank you so much. We really appreciate your help.

**病人家属**:谢谢,真的非常感谢你们的帮助。

## Useful Expressions

Were there any special conditions when the baby was born?

新生儿出生的时候有没有什么异常的情况?

Was the baby moving or crying?

新生儿有没有动或者是哭?

Did the baby seem to have difficulty breathing?

新生儿是否呼吸困难?

Can you please tell me if the baby was born full-term or premature?

您能告诉我新生儿是足月出生还是早产吗?

Were there any complications during pregnancy or labor?

孕期或生产时有没有出现并发症?

> **Q Key Words and Phrases**
>
> **pregnancy** ['pregnənsi] n. 怀孕,妊娠
> **labor** ['leibə] n. 分娩

Was there a prolonged labor?

分娩持续时间是否较长？

Was there a premature rupture of membranes?

是否胎膜早破？

Are there seizures?

是否有癫痫发作？

Does the baby seem floppy or stiff?

新生儿看起来是否身体软弱或僵硬？

I'll perform a quick assessment of the baby's responsiveness, breathing, and color.

我现在要进行新生儿反应、呼吸和颜色的快速评估。

I'm going to clear any mucus or other obstructions from the baby's airway.

我要清除一下新生儿气道中的黏液或其他分泌物。

I am going to administer oxygen to the baby and gently stimulate him / her to breathe.

我会为新生儿提供氧气，并轻柔地刺激他 / 她呼吸。

We're going to transport him / her to the hospital right away for further treatment.

我们现在要尽快将他 / 她转送到医院进行进一步治疗。

The baby appears stable but still at risk due to suspected asphyxia at birth.

新生儿现在情况稳定，但由

于出生时疑似出现窒息,所以还存在一定的风险。

## Section 2　Apnea of Prematurity
## 早产儿呼吸暂停

### Conversation

Patient, male, 3 weeks old, was premature infant who was born at 28 weeks gestation weighing 2.2 kg. He was discharged home from the NICU one week ago. This morning, his family members noticed him turning blue and unresponsive. They called for emergency medical services.

患儿,男性,3 周,是 28 周胎龄时出生的早产儿,出生时体重 2.2kg。1 周前从新生儿重症监护室出院回家。今天早上,家属发现新生儿面色发青,呼之不应,他们拨打了 120 急救电话。

**Doctor:** Hello, I'm Dr. Han. We got a call for help here. Can you tell me what happened?

医生:您好! 我是韩医生。我们接到了急救电话,您能告诉我发生了什么事吗?

---

**Q Key Words and Phrases**

**apnea** ['æpnɪə] n. 呼吸暂停,无呼吸,窒息

**prematurity** [pri:mə'tjʊrətɪ] n. 早产儿,早熟

**gestation** [dʒe'steɪʃn] n. 怀孕,怀孕期

**discharge** [dɪs'tʃɑ:dʒ] v. 允许……离开

**NICU** (neonatal intensive care unit 的简称) 新生儿重症监护病房

**Patient's family member:** It's my 3-week-old son. He was born prematurely at 28 weeks and has been home from the NICU for a week now. This morning I went to check on him and he was turning blue and not responding at all.

病人家属：是我 3 周大的孩子需要帮助。他在胎龄 28 周时早产，一周前才从新生儿重症监护室出院回家。今天早上我去看他的时候，发现他脸色发青，呼之不应。

**Doctor:** OK, I understand. Can I take a look at him?

医生：好的，了解。我现在可以看看他吗？

**Patient's family member:** Yes, of course! He's not breathing normally and his lips are still blue. I'm so worried!

病人家属：当然。他的呼吸很不规律，嘴唇也发青，我真的很担心。

**Doctor:** All right, we're going to take good care of him. Now I am going to perform a quick assessment of him. Let me know if you have questions.

医生：别担心，我们会照顾好他的。现在我要为他做一个快速评估，要是有什么问题您可以随时提问。

*After assessment, the doctor finds the baby has a weak pulse, low heart rate (below 100 beats/min), and a purple face and lips.*

*经过评估，医生发现新生儿脉搏微弱、心率偏低（低于 100 次 /min），面部、嘴唇发紫。*

**Doctor:** Were there any special situations before your baby had difficulty breathing, like spitting up or vomiting?

医生：新生儿出现呼吸困

难前有没有什么异常情况发生？比如呛奶、呕吐等。

**Patient's family member:** No, everything was normal.

病人家属：没有什么特别的情况发生。

**Doctor:** Did the baby have any diseases that could induce apnea, such as respiratory system diseases, <u>congenital</u> heart disease, or infectious diseases?

医生：新生儿是否患有可能会诱发呼吸暂停的疾病？比如呼吸系统疾病、先天性心脏病或感染性疾病。

**Patient's family member:** No. He stayed in NICU for low weight, but everything was fine then.

病人家属：没有。他之前因为体重偏低住进了新生儿重症监护室，但那时一切都很正常。

**Doctor:** We suspect that he has apnea of prematurity. We'll get him to the hospital as quickly and safely as we can. I'm going to clear his airway and put an oxygen mask on him to help him breathe a bit easier. Then we'll get him on a monitor and start an intravenous infusion.

医生：我们怀疑他是早产儿呼吸暂停。我们现在会尽快将他安全转送到医院。我会先清理他的呼吸道，给他戴上氧气面罩，让他呼吸得更顺畅些。然后我们会给他接上监护仪，并开始静脉输液。

**Patient's family member:** Thank you so much. Please take good care of my son.

病人家属：谢谢您，医生，请一定帮忙照顾好我的儿子。

---

🔍 **Key Words and Phrases**

**congenital** [kənˈdʒenɪtl] adj. 先天的，天生的

## Useful Expressions

Now I am going to perform a quick assessment of the baby.

现在我要为新生儿做一个快速评估。

Were there any special situations before your baby had difficulty breathing, like spitting up or vomiting?

新生儿出现呼吸困难前有没有什么异常情况发生？比如呛奶、呕吐等。

Did the baby have any diseases that could induce apnea, such as respiratory system diseases, congenital heart disease or infectious diseases?

新生儿是否患有可能会诱发呼吸暂停的疾病？比如呼吸系统疾病、先天性心脏病或感染性疾病。

How frequently are the apnea episodes occurring?

呼吸暂停发作的频率如何？

Has the baby received any medications or treatments for the apnea?

新生儿是否服用过治疗呼吸暂停的药物或接受过相关治疗？

Other than the breathing stops, has the baby had any choking, turning blue, or required resuscitation?

除了呼吸停止之外，新生儿是否有过窒息、皮肤发紫或者需要复苏的情况？

Given the prematurity, apnea is likely. We need to

**Key Words and Phrases**

choke [ˈtʃəʊk] v.（使）窒息
resuscitation [rɪˌsʌsɪˈteɪʃn] n. 恢复知觉，苏醒

support his / her breathing right away.

考虑到是早产儿,非常可能是呼吸暂停发作,我们现在需要立刻辅助他 / 她进行呼吸。

I'm going to suction his / her airway and put an oxygen mask on him / her to help him / her breathe a bit easier.

我会先清理他 / 她的呼吸道,给他 / 她戴上氧气面罩,让他 / 她呼吸得更顺畅些。

We may need to intubate if he / she has further apnea episodes on the way to the hospital.

如果他 / 她在去医院的路上再次发生呼吸暂停,我们可能需要为他 / 她插管。

We'll continue monitoring his / her breathing, oxygen levels, and heart rate for any signs of apnea.

我们会继续监测他 / 她的呼吸、血氧和心率,观察是否有呼吸暂停的迹象。

## Section 3　Febrile Convulsion
## 高热惊厥

### Conversation

**Patient, male, 3 years old, developed a high fever with no apparent cause about an hour ago. His temperature rose as high as 38.8°C, and he subsequently became disoriented, had convulsion**

🔍 **Key Words and Phrases**

**intubate** [ˈɪntjʊbeɪt] v. 把管子插进

**febrile** [ˈfiːbraɪl] adj. 发热的

**convulsion** [kənˈvʌlʃən] n. 抽搐

**disoriented** [dɪˈsɔːrɪəntɪd] adj. 无判断力的

**in all four limbs, rolled his eyes, and his face turned blue. These symptoms lasted for about a minute and gradually disappeared. His family member called for emergency medical services.**

患儿,男性,3 岁,1 小时前无明显诱因出现高热,体温最高达 38.8℃,随即出现意识不清、四肢抽搐、双眼上翻、面色青紫,持续 1 分钟左右后逐渐缓解,家属拨打了 120 急救电话。

**Doctor:** Hello, I'm Dr. Han. What seems to be the problem?

医生:您好,我是韩医生。请问发生了什么事?

**Patient's family member:** Something is wrong with our son. He is three years old. He developed a high fever about an hour ago for unknown reason. His temperature went up to 38.8 degrees <u>Celsius</u> and then he started having convulsion, rolling his eyes and his face turned blue.

病人家属:我的儿子不太舒服,他 3 岁了,1 小时前不知道怎么回事突然发高烧,体温最高达到了 38.8℃,然后他突然开始抽搐,两眼上翻,脸色发青。

**Doctor:** OK, try to stay calm. This sounds like a febrile convulsion caused by the high fever. How is he doing now?

医生:好的,请尽量保持冷静。可能是高热引起的高热惊厥。他现在怎么样了?

**Patient's family member:** The convulsion stopped after about a minute. But I'm really worried.

病人家属:抽搐持续了差不多 1 分钟就停止了。但是我真的很担心。

> 🔍 **Key Words and Phrases**
>
> **Celsius** [ˈselsiəs] n. 摄氏度

**Doctor:** I understand your concern. Did he vomit during the seizures?

医生:我理解您的担心。他在发作过程中有没有呕吐?

**Patient's family member:** Yes, a little. And this is the first time that he had such a convulsion.

病人家属:吐了一点点。这也是他第一次出现抽搐。

**Doctor:** Got it. Now we need to let him lie on his side to prevent aspiration of vomit. And my colleague is going to check his vitals.

医生:了解。我们要让他保持侧卧,防止误吸呕吐物。我的同事会检查他的生命体征。

*The nurse checks the child's temperature, pulse, breathing and wrap a piece of gauze around a tongue depressor and places it between the upper and lower molars to prevent biting of the tongue.*

*护士检查了患儿的体温、脉搏、呼吸,并用纱布包裹压舌板,置于上下磨牙之间,防止幼儿咬伤舌头。*

**Nurse:** When a seizure happens, please try to stay calm and do not shout at or shake the child. Now his temperature is still high but the convulsion have stopped. We need to bring the fever down to prevent another seizure.

护士:如果发生惊厥,请尽量保持冷静,不要大喊大叫,或者摇晃孩子。他现在体温还是比较高,但已经不抽搐了。我们必须尽快让体温降下来,防止再

---

🔍 **Key Words and Phrases**

**gauze** [ɡɔːz] n. 纱布(包扎伤口用)

**depressor** [dɪˈpresə(r)] n. (检验或手术中用的)压板

**molar** [məʊˈlə] n. 磨牙

---

次发作。

**Patient's family member:** What should we do?

病人家属：我们应该怎么做?

**Doctor:** Try to keep your child cool by removing any excess clothing and covering him with a light sheet.

医生：尽量给患儿降温，可以脱掉多余的衣物，覆盖轻薄的被子。

**Patient's family member:** OK, thank you.

病人家属：好的，谢谢。

**Doctor:** Now I am going to put an oxygen mask on him to help him breathe a bit easier and start an intravenous injection to control the seizure. Let's get him to the ambulance, and we need to transport him to the hospital for further examination.

医生：我现在要给他戴上氧气面罩，让他呼吸得更顺畅些，同时给予静脉注射来控制惊厥。让我们把他抬上救护车，送往医院进行进一步检查。

**Patient's family member:** That's reassuring. Thank you for the quick response. I'm riding with him in the ambulance, right?

病人家属：这样我们就安心多了，谢谢你们的及时救助。我是要跟着救护车一起走，对吧?

**Doctor:** Yes, you can accompany us to the hospital. We will continue to monitor his vitals and I'll explain what's happening during the trip and answer any other questions you have.

医生：对，您可以跟车一起去医院。我们会继续监测他的生命体征，途中我会向您解释发生了什么，您要是有什么疑惑，也可以随时问我们。

**Patient's family member:** OK, thank you for your help.

病人家属：好的，感谢你们的帮助。

## Useful Expressions

Let me take your child's vitals to assess the fever.

让我测量一下您孩子的生命体征以评估发热情况。

Did he / she vomit during the seizures?

他 / 她在发作过程中有没有呕吐？

Let him / her lie on his / her side to prevent aspiration of vomit.

让他 / 她保持侧卧，防止误吸呕吐物。

Can you describe to me what the seizure looked like and how long it lasted?

您能描述一下发作的情况和持续了多久吗？

Was this your child's first seizure or have there been episodes in the past?

这是您孩子第一次发作还是以前也有过？

It appears your child had a simple febrile convulsion brought on by the high fever. These are common in children.

您的孩子似乎是因为高热引起了简单高热惊厥，这在儿童中很常见。

When a seizure happens, please try to stay calm and do not shout at or shake the child.

如果发生惊厥，请尽量保持冷静，不要大喊大叫，或者摇晃患儿。

Try to keep your child cool by removing any excess clothing

and covering him with a light sheet.

尽量给患儿降温, 可以脱掉多余的衣物, 盖轻薄的被子。

Make sure to keep the fever down with acetaminophen / ibuprofen.

可以服用对乙酰氨基酚或布洛芬以确保退烧。

I am going to put an oxygen mask on him / her to help him / her breathe a bit easier.

我现在要给他 / 她戴上氧气面罩, 让他 / 她呼吸得更顺畅些。

I will monitor his / her cardiac rhythm with electrocardiogram monitor and observe for any arrhythmias.

我会用心电监护仪对他 / 她进行心电监护, 观察是否有心律失常。

If necessary, we will start an intravenous injection to prevent dehydration or another seizure.

有必要的话, 我们还会给予静脉注射以防止脱水或再次惊厥发作。

---

🔍 **Key Words and Phrases**

**acetaminophen** [əˌsiːtəˈmɪnəfen] n. 对乙酰氨基酚

**ibuprofen** [ˌaɪbjuːˈprəʊfen] n. 布洛芬, 异丁苯丙酸

**cardiac rhythm** 心律

**arrhythmia** [əˈrɪðmiːə] n. <内科> 心律失常, 心律不整

# Unit 4

## Common Injuries Caused by Environmental and Physicochemical Factors
## 环境及理化因素所致常见损伤

### Section 1　Heat Stroke
### 中暑

#### Conversation

Patient, male, 60 years old, experienced severe symptoms such as sweating all over, nausea, dizziness, blurred vision, weak limbs, and dry mouth. His family member called for emergency medical services.

病人,男性,60 岁,出现全身出汗、恶心、头晕、眼花、四肢无力、口干等严重症状,家属拨打了 120 急救电话。

**Doctor:** Hello, I'm Li Hua, an EMT. Can you tell me what happened?

医生:您好! 我叫李华,是一名急救医生,您能告诉我发生了什么事吗?

**Patient's family member:** It's my father, Mr. Zhang. He is 60 years old. This afternoon, he was working in our garden. When he came inside, he didn't seem well.

**病人家属:**是我父亲,张先生,他已经60岁了。今天中午,他在花园里干活儿,当他回屋子里的时候,他看上去很不舒服。

**Doctor:** Has the patient been exposed to high temperatures or spent time in the sun?

**医生:**病人是不是暴露在了高温环境中或者在太阳下待了很长时间?

**Patient's family member:** Yes, it was quite hot, and he's been in the garden for about an hour.

**病人家属:**对,天气挺热的,他在花园里待了差不多一个小时。

**Doctor:** Can you tell me what symptoms the patient has been experiencing?

**医生:**您能告诉我病人都有哪些症状吗?

**Patient's family member:** Yes, he was sweating heavily and felt unwell. He said he felt nauseous, dizzy, and his vision was blurred.

**病人家属:**他流了很多的汗,觉得不舒服,他说他感觉恶心、头晕,而且视物模糊。

**Doctor:** Did he mention any other symptoms?

**医生:**他还提到了其他症状吗?

---

🔍 **Key Words and Phrases**

**be exposed to** 暴露于,暴露在,面临

**Patient's family member:** Yes, he also said his mouth was dry and he felt weakness in his arms and legs.

病人家属：有，他还说他的嘴巴很干，四肢无力。

**Doctor:** Those symptoms sound like a heat stroke. Let me check his temperature and blood pressure.

医生：这些听起来像是中暑的症状。让我量一下他的体温和血压。

*After examination, the doctor turns to the patient and asks questions.*

*检查后，医生转向病人并提问。*

**Doctor:** Mr. Zhang, Can you hear me? Can you tell me what happened?

医生：张先生，您能听到我说话吗，您能告诉我发生了什么事吗？

*Mr. Zhang doesn't respond and starts experiencing delirium, convulsion, incoherent speech and other symptoms.*

*张先生没有回应，并开始出现精神错乱、抽搐、言语不清等症状。*

**Doctor:** He seems to have severe heat stroke. He's been exhibiting signs like high body temperature, rapid pulse, confusion and possible loss of consciousness. We need to lower his temperature quickly and get fluids into him. Has the patient been drinking enough water?

医生：他看起来中暑非常严重。他已经出现了体温过高、脉搏过快、意识

**🔍 Key Words and Phrases**

**delirium** [dɪˈlɪriəm] n. 精神错乱，神志昏迷，极度兴奋

· 165 ·

不清的症状,且可能失去了知觉。我们需要尽快为他降温和补液。病人饮水量是否充足?

**Patient's family member:** No, he said he felt too sick to drink.

病人家属:没有,他说他特别不舒服,喝不下。

**Doctor:** We need to lower his temperature immediately. I will remove his shirt to expose more skin and <u>spray</u> him with cold water.

医生:我们需要立即降低他的体温。我需要脱掉他的衬衫,让更多的皮肤暴露在外面,然后用冷水淋他。

**Patient's family member:** Alright, we'll help. Does he need to drink water?

病人家属:好的,我们来一起帮忙。需要给他喝点水吗?

**Doctor:** Yes, please use ice water to <u>moisten</u> his lips and gently let him drink a little.

医生:是的,请用冰水帮他润润嘴唇,让他慢慢地喝一点儿水。

**Patient's family member:** OK.

病人家属:好的。

**Doctor:** We need to transport him to the hospital as soon as possible. I'm going to place ice packs in his <u>armpits</u> and <u>groin</u> to start cooling him on the way. Please help me get him onto the stretcher.

医生:我们需要尽快将他送到医院去。我现在要在他的腋

| 🔍 **Key Words and Phrases** |
| --- |
| **spray** [spreɪ] v. 喷 |
| **moisten** [ˈmɔɪsn] v. (使)变得潮湿 |
| **armpit** [ˈɑːmˌpɪt] n. 腋窝 |
| **groin** [grɔɪn] n. 腹股沟,交叉拱,穹窿交接线,堤坝 |

下和腹股沟处放一些冰袋,在途中降低他的体温。请帮助我们
把您父亲抬到担架上。

*The patient is transferred to the ambulance.*

*病人被送到了救护车上。*

**Doctor:** Now I am going to check his vital signs and my
partner will get some intravenous injection fluids ready, and this
will provide the fluids and electrolytes he needs. And we will put
an oxygen mask on him to help him breathe more easily.

医生:现在,我要检查他的生命体征,我的同事会为他预备
静脉输液,这可以为他提供需要的液体和电解质。我们还会给
他戴上氧气面罩,让他呼吸得更顺畅些。

**Patient's family member:** Thank you so much. Please take
good care of him!

病人家属:谢谢,请帮助照顾好我的父亲!

**Doctor:** Don't worry. We'll continue aggressively cooling
him and replenishing his fluids and monitor him closely.

医生:别担心,我们会继续积极地帮他降温和补充液体,也
会密切监测。

## Useful Expressions

Has the patient been exposed to high temperatures or spent
time in the sun?

病人是不是暴露在了高温环境中或者太阳下待了很长
时间?

Can you tell me what symptoms the patient has been
experiencing?

您能描述一下病人的症状吗?

Those symptoms sound like a heat stroke.

这些听起来都像是中暑的症状。

Let's check his / her temperature and blood pressure.

让我量一下他 / 她的体温和血压。

I'm going to examine him / her for signs of dehydration.

我要检查他 / 她是否出现了脱水的迹象。

He's / She's exhibiting signs of heat stroke like high body temperature, rapid pulse, confusion and loss of consciousness.

他 / 她出现了中暑的症状,如体温过高、脉搏加快、意识混乱以及失去知觉。

Has the patient been drinking enough water?

病人饮水量是否充足?

We need to lower the patient's body temperature as quickly as possible to prevent further damage.

我们需要尽快降低病人的体温,防止进一步的伤害。

We'll need to remove any excess clothing and use ice packs in the patient's armpits, groin and neck to help cool him / her down.

我们需要脱掉病人多余的衣物,并在他 / 她的腋下、腹股沟和颈部放置冰袋来帮助降温。

Dehydration makes heat stroke worse, so we need to get some fluids into the patient.

脱水会加重中暑,所以我们需要为病人补充体液。

If physical cooling methods don't reduce the patient's temperature soon, we may consider giving intravenous injection fluids or medication to control fever.

如果物理降温方法不能很快地降低病人的体温,我们可能会考虑给予静脉输液或药物来控制发热。

The patient may need to be hospitalized for treatment and monitoring.

病人可能需要住院治疗和监测。

It's important to rest and avoid heat exposure until the patient is fully recovered.

在病人完全恢复之前,一定要好好休息,避免暴露在高温环境中。

# Section 2　Drowning
# 淹溺

## Conversation

**Patient, male, 10 years old, accidentally fell into a lake. Several adult men jumped into the lake to rescue him and a witness called for emergency medical services.**

患儿,男性,10 岁,失足落入湖中,几名成年男子跳入湖中将其救出,一名目击者拨打了 120 急救电话。

**Doctor:** Hello, I'm Dr. Han. Can you tell me what happened?

医生:您好,我是韩医生。您能告诉我发生了什么事吗?

**Witness:** Yes, a 10-year-old boy was having a picnic with his parents in a park. He accidentally fell into the lake while his parents

> **Q Key Words and Phrases**
>
> **drowning** [draʊnɪŋ] n. 溺水
> **rescue** [ˈreskjuː] v. 营救

were preparing lunch. Some of us jumped in and pulled him out of the water.

**目击者:** 好的, 一个 10 岁的男孩和他父母在公园里野餐。他父母准备午餐的时候, 他不小心掉进湖里了。我们有人跳进湖里, 把他拉了上来。

**Doctor:** How long was he under water before you pulled him out?

**医生:** 在你们把他拉出水面之前, 他在水下待了多长时间?

**Witness:** I think around 3 minutes. As soon as we heard the <u>splash</u> and <u>yelling</u>, we ran over to help.

**目击者:** 大概 3 分钟。我们一听到溅水声和呼救声, 就立即跑过去帮忙了。

**Doctor:** Did the patient lose consciousness at any point?

**医生:** 病人有没有失去过知觉?

**Witness:** Yes, he has lost consciousness. One of the men did cardiopulmonary resuscitation on him after we got him out of the water. And he regained his consciousness gradually. But his breathing seems very faint now.

**目击者:** 有的, 他当时已经失去知觉了。有人在我们把他从水中救出来后, 对他进行了心肺复苏, 然后他慢慢恢复了意识, 但是他的呼吸现在非常微弱。

**Doctor:** Did he cough up any water?

**医生:** 他有咳出水来吗?

**Witness:** He coughed up some water initially after being rescued.

**Key Words and Phrases**

**splash** [splæʃ] n. 溅泼声
**yelling** [jeliŋ] n. 大声喊

**目击者:**刚被救起来的时候,他咳出了一些水。

**Doctor:** OK, we'll take over now. Please make room for us.

**医生:**好的,我们现在来接手。请为我们让出空间。

*The doctor checks the boy immediately and asks questions.*

*医生迅速对男孩进行了检查,并提问。*

**Doctor:** Can you hear me? What's your name and age?

**医生:**你能听到我说话吗,你叫什么名字,多大了?

*The patient mumbles.*

*病人言语不清。*

**Patient's family member:** His name is Jack. He's 10 years old.

**病人家属:**他叫杰克,今年 10 岁。

**Doctor:** Does he have any chronic illnesses such as asthma or heart disease?

**医生:**他是否患有哮喘、心脏病等慢性疾病?

**Patient's family member:** No, he has always been very healthy.

**病人家属:**没有,他的身体一直都很健康。

**Doctor:** Has he had any recent medical conditions or surgeries?

**医生:**他最近生过病或做过手术吗?

**Patient's family member:** No.

**病人家属:**没有。

**Doctor:** Does he have a history of medication allergies?

**医生:**他有药物过敏史吗?

**Patient's family member:** No.

**病人家属:**没有。

> 🔍 **Key Words and Phrases**
>
> **mumble** ['mʌmbl] v. 叽咕,咕哝

**Doctor:** OK, we are going to transfer him to the ambulance and get some oxygen on. Please ride with us to the hospital.

医生：我们现在要把他送到救护车上，给他吸氧，请您跟着我们的救护车一起去医院。

**Patient's family member:** Yes, of course. Thank you so much. Will he be OK?

病人家属：好的，非常感谢。他会没事的吧？

**Doctor:** My partner is putting him on oxygen now and starting an intravenous injection. And we will monitor him closely through the electrocardiogram all the way to the hospital. The doctors will take good care of him.

医生：我的搭档现在给他吸氧，准备静脉注射。在去医院的路上，我们会通过心电监护密切观察他的情况，医院的医生会照顾好他的。

**Patient's family member:** OK, thank you very much. Please help him.

病人家属：好的，非常感谢。请一定要救救他。

## Useful Expressions

*For the witness:*

*向目击者提问：*

How long was the patient under water before you pulled him / her out?

在你们把他／她拉出水面之前，病人在水下待了多长时间？

Did the patient lose consciousness at any point?

病人有没有失去过知觉？

Did the patient cough up any water?

病人有没有咳出水来？

**For the patient:**

*向病人提问：*

Can you hear me? What's your name and age?

您能听到我说话吗，您叫什么名字，多少岁了？

**For the family member:**

*向家属提问：*

Does he / she have any chronic illnesses such as asthma or heart disease?

他／她是否患有哮喘、心脏病等慢性疾病？

Has he / she had any recent medical conditions or surgeries?

他／她最近生过病或做过手术吗？

Does he / she have a history of medication allergies?

他／她有药物过敏史吗？

We will put the patient on oxygen now and start an intravenous injection.

我们现在给病人吸氧，准备静脉注射。

We will monitor the patient closely through the electrocardiogram.

我们将通过心电监护密切观察病人的情况。

We need to get the patient to the hospital for further evaluation and treatment.

我们需要将病人送往医院，进行进一步评估和治疗。

# Section 3　Electric Shock
# 触电

## Conversation

Patient, male, 35 years old, was <u>electrocuted</u> and fell down while repairing <u>electrical</u> <u>appliances</u> at home. His family member immediately called for emergency medical services.

病人,男性,35 岁,在家修理电器时,不慎触电倒地,家属立即拨打了 120 急救电话。

**Doctor:** Hi, I'm Li Hua, a paramedic. Can you tell me what happened?

医生:您好,我叫李华,是一名急救医生。您能告诉我发生了什么事吗?

**Patient's family member:** It's my brother. He was trying to fix an electrical appliance at home, but suddenly he got electrocuted. He fell down to the ground and now he has lost consciousness. He's not breathing and we can't feel his pulse.

病人家属:是我哥哥,他在家里修理电器时,突然触电了,他倒在地上,失去了意识,也没有呼吸和脉搏。

**Doctor:** OK, did you <u>cut off</u> the power?

医生:了解,你们切断电源了吗?

**Patient's family member:**

🔍 **Key Words and Phrases**

**electrocute** [ilektrəkjuːt] v. 触电

**electrical** [ɪˈlektrɪkl] adj. 用电的

**appliance** [əˈplaɪəns] n. 器具

**cut off** 切除

Yes, we cut off the power immediately after the accident.

病人家属:事故发生之后我们立刻切断了电源。

**Doctor:** Did anyone perform cardiopulmonary resuscitation on him?

医生:有人给他进行过心肺复苏吗?

**Patient's family member:** No, we didn't know how to do it.

病人家属:没有,我们都不知道怎么操作。

**Doctor:** Alright, don't worry. We'll take care of him. We need to start cardiopulmonary resuscitation immediately to try to revive him. I'll perform chest compressions while my partner sets up the defibrillator.

医生:好的,不用担心。我们会照顾他的。我们需要立即开始心肺复苏,让他苏醒过来。我来进行胸外心脏按压,我的搭档会准备好除颤器。

**Patient's family member:** Is he going to be OK?

病人家属:他会没事的吧?

**Doctor:** We'll do everything we can to help him. It's important that we act quickly in situations like this.

医生:我们会尽力帮助他。在这种情况下,迅速行动非常重要。

*Doctor and nurse begin to do the cardiopulmonary resuscitation and use the defibrillator. After several minutes, the patient regains a pulse and starts breathing again.*

急救人员开始进行心肺复苏术并使用除颤器。几分钟

**Key Words and Phrases**

revive [rɪˈvaɪv] v. 使复活
regain [riˈɡeɪn] v. 恢复

*后,病人恢复了脉搏和呼吸。*

**Doctor:** OK, his pulse is back. But he has obvious skin burns, swelling around the wound, and some slight bleeding. We need to administer pain relief treatment and clean the wound to prevent infection.

医生:好的,他的脉搏恢复了。但是他的伤口附近有明显的皮肤烧伤和肿胀,同时有些许出血。我们要对他进行止痛治疗,并清洁伤口,以避免感染。

*The nurse cleans the wound and provides pain relief treatment.*
*护士清理了病人的伤口,并给予止痛治疗。*

**Doctor:** We're going to take him to the hospital for further treatment. He's still in critical condition.

医生:我们要把他送到医院进行进一步治疗。他仍处于危急状态。

**Patient's family member:** Thank you so much for your help.

病人家属:谢谢你们的帮助。

## Useful Expressions

Can you tell me exactly what happened and how did the patient get shocked?

您能告诉我具体发生了什么事吗,病人是怎么触电的?

Did you cut off the power?

你们切断电源了吗?

Did anyone perform cardiopulmonary resuscitation on the patient?

有人给病人进行过心肺复苏吗?

Let's start cardiopulmonary resuscitation. I'll perform chest compressions while my partner sets up the defibrillator.

我们开始心肺复苏。我来进行胸外心脏按压,我的搭档会准备好除颤器。

We need to run some tests to assess the extent of the damage.

我们需要进行一些测试来评估损伤的程度。

The patient has obvious skin burns, swelling around the wound, and some slight bleeding.

病人的伤口附近有明显的皮肤烧伤和肿胀,同时有些许出血。

We need to administer pain relief treatment and clean the wound to prevent infection.

我们要对他进行止痛治疗,并清洁伤口,以避免感染。

The patient may be at risk for complications such as muscle damage or kidney failure.

病人可能面临发生肌肉损伤或肾功能衰竭等并发症的风险。

We need to assess the patient's heart function with an electrocardiogram.

我们需要通过心电图评估病人的心脏功能。

We need to check for any internal injuries, such as damage to organs or tissues.

我们需要检查是否有内部损伤,比如器官或组织的损伤。

It's important to avoid further exposure to electrical currents to prevent further injury.

> **🔍 Key Words and Phrases**
>
> **internal injury** 内部损伤,内伤
>
> **electrical current** 电流

重要的是，要避免进一步接触电流，以防止进一步受伤。

# Section 4　Burns and Scalds
# 烧烫伤

## 1. Scald Caused by Hot Liquid 热液烫伤

## Conversation

**Patient, female, 32 years old, scalded both forearms and hands with boiling water while cooking two hours ago. She called for emergency medical services.**

病人，女性，32 岁，2 小时前，做饭时被开水烫伤双前臂和双手，她拨打了 120 急救电话。

**Doctor:** Hello, I'm one of the doctors who responded to your call. Can you tell me what happened?

医生：您好，我是 120 急救医生，您能告诉我发生了什么事吗？

**Patient:** Yes, I was cooking and accidentally spilled boiling water on my forearms and hands. It really hurts.

病人：好的，我当时正在做饭，不小心被开水溅到了我的前臂和手上，真的很痛。

**Doctor:** I'm sorry to hear that. Let's take a look at your injuries.

医生：很抱歉听到您遇到

> **Q Key Words and Phrases**
>
> **scald** [skɔːld] n. (沸水或蒸汽造成的) 烫伤

了这样的事。让我来检查一下您的伤口。

*The doctor examines the scalds.*

医生检查烫伤部位。

**Doctor:** The scalds look deep and severe. We need to cool them down immediately.

医生：伤口看起来很深，比较严重，我们需要立刻给伤口降温。

**Patient:** OK, please help me.

病人：好的，请帮帮我。

**Doctor:** We'll start by flushing the scalds with cool water for at least 10 minutes.

医生：我们将用凉水冲洗伤口至少10分钟。

*The doctor starts flushing the scald with cool water.*

医生开始用凉水冲洗伤口。

**Doctor:** How long ago did this happen?

医生：这是什么时候发生的事？

**Patient:** About two hours ago.

病人：大约2小时前。

**Doctor:** Do you feel any numbness in the affected area?

医生：烫伤部位有没有感觉发麻？

**Patient:** A little bit.

病人：有一点儿。

**Doctor:** Can you move your fingers and wrists?

医生：您能动一下您的手指和手腕吗？

*The patient moves her fingers*

🔍 **Key Words and Phrases**

**flush** [ˈflʌʃ] v. 冲刷

*and wrists slowly.*

病人慢慢动了动手指和手腕。

**Doctor:** Let me check if there is any redness or swelling around the scalds.

医生：我检查一下烫伤部位有没有红肿。

*After examining the wounds.*

检查之后。

**Doctor:** Have you taken any pain medication or applied any ointment to the scalds?

医生：您有没有服用止痛药或者在烫伤处涂抹药膏？

**Patient:** No.

病人：没有。

**Doctor:** OK, we need to get you to the hospital for further treatment. The scalds could cause infection and other complications if not treated promptly.

医生：好的，我们需要将您送往医院进行进一步治疗。如果不及时治疗，烫伤可能会引发感染和其他并发症。

**Patient:** OK, I understand.

病人：好的，了解。

**Doctor:** We'll wrap your scalds in a sterile dressing to protect them and provide pain relief. Please try to keep your hands

---

🔍 **Key Words and Phrases**

**ointment** [ˈɔɪntmənt] n. 软膏，药膏，油膏

**sterile** [ˈsteraɪl] adj. 无菌的，不生育的

**dressing** [ˈdresɪŋ] n. 敷料

**pain relief** 减轻或消除疼痛的方法或药物，止痛

elevated to reduce swelling.

病人：为了保护您的伤口，我们将用无菌敷料进行包扎。同时我们会给您一些止痛药。请尽量保持手部抬高，以消除肿胀。

**Patient:** Thank you so much for your help.

病人：谢谢你们的帮助。

**Doctor:** You're welcome. We'll provide the best care possible. Let's get you to the hospital now.

医生：不用谢，我们将尽一切努力为您提供最佳护理。现在让我们把您送到医院。

## Useful Expressions

Can you tell me how the scald happened?

您能告诉我您是怎么烫伤的吗？

How long ago did the scald happen?

是什么时候烫伤的？

We'll start by flushing the scalds with cool water.

我们将用凉水冲洗烫伤伤口。

Do you feel any numbness in the affected area?

烫伤部位有没有感觉发麻？

Can you move your fingers and wrists?

您能动一下您的手指和手腕吗？

Let me check if there is any redness or swelling around the scalds.

我检查一下烫伤部位有没有红肿。

> **Key Words and Phrases**
>
> **elevate** [ˈelɪveɪt] v. 举起

Have you taken any pain medication or applied any ointment to the scalds?

您有没有服用止痛药或者在烫伤处涂抹药膏？

Let me check the color and texture of the blister.

我给您检查一下水疱的颜色和质地。

We'll wrap your scalds in a sterile dressing to protect them and provide pain relief.

为了保护您的伤口，我们将用无菌敷料进行包扎。同时我们会给您一些止痛药。

Please try to keep your hands elevated to reduce swelling.

请尽量保持手部抬高，以消除肿胀。

The scalds could cause infection and other complications if not treated promptly.

如果不及时治疗，烫伤可能会引发感染和其他并发症。

## 2. Contact Burn 接触性烫伤

## Conversation

**Patient, male, 60 years old, accidentally got burnt while using an electric blanket to keep himself warm during cold weather. His family member called for emergency medical services.**

病人，男性，60 岁，因天气寒冷使用电热毯保暖，不慎被烫伤，家属拨打了 120 急救电话。

> 🔍 **Key Words and Phrases**
>
> **electric blanket** 电热毯

**Doctor:** Hello sir, can you hear me?

医生：您好，先生，您能听见我说话吗？

**Patient:** Yes, I can hear you.

病人：是的，我听得到。

**Doctor:** I'm a doctor, and I'm here to help you. Can you tell me how you got this burn?

医生：我是一名急救医生，是来帮助您的。您能告诉我您是怎么被烫伤的吗？

**Patient:** I felt so cold last night that I used my electric blanket to keep myself warm. But I guess I fell asleep and forgot to turn it off. When I woke up this morning, I got burnt and I had blisters on both my hands and feet.

病人：昨晚我觉得太冷了，就打开了电热毯保暖。但是我可能是睡着的时候忘记关掉它了，早上我起来的时候，就发现被烫伤了，我的手脚上都起了水疱。

**Doctor:** I see. Where exactly is the burn located?

医生：明白了，具体烫伤部位在哪里？

**Patient:** They're on my hands and feet.

病人：就在我的手和脚上。

**Doctor:** On a scale of 1 to 10, with 10 being the worst, how would you rate your pain from the burn?

医生：用 1 到 10 分来评估，10 分为最痛，您会给您的烫伤疼痛程度打几分？

**Patient:** Maybe 8 or 9. It really hurts.

病人：大概 8 分或 9 分吧。真的很痛。

**Doctor:** OK, I'm going to examine them now.

医生:好的,我现在检查一下。

*The doctor examins the burns.*

医生检查烫伤部位。

**Doctor:** It looks like you have second-degree burns with blisters. We need to <u>cool down</u> the burns right away to prevent further damage. Can you tell me if you have any allergies or medical conditions?

医生:看起来您属于Ⅱ度烫伤,有水疱出现。我们需要尽快降温,防止进一步的感染。请问您有过敏史或疾病史吗?

**Patient:** No, I don't have any allergies or medical conditions.

病人:没有,我没有过敏或疾病史。

**Doctor:** OK, I'm going to start by cleaning the burns with cold water and applying a sterile dressing. This will help to reduce the pain and prevent infection. How are you feeling otherwise? Any dizziness, nausea?

医生:好的,我现在要用冷水清洗烫伤部位,并敷上无菌敷料,这有助于减轻疼痛并预防感染。您其他方面感觉如何,有眩晕和恶心吗?

**Patient:** A bit dizzy but no nausea. Just a lot of pain in my hands and feet.

病人:有点晕,但是不恶心。只是我的手和脚很痛。

**Doctor:** The pain is normal, burns often cause severe pain. I'll give you some pain relief medications to help you feel more comfortable.

医生:痛是正常的,烧烫伤通常会引起剧烈疼痛。我会给

---

🔍 **Key Words and Phrases**

**cool down**（使）变凉

---

您一些止痛药物,让您感觉舒服些。

**Patient:** Thank you.

病人:谢谢。

**Doctor:** It's important that you avoid touching or scratching the blisters, as it can cause them to burst and become infected. You should also avoid exposing the burns to heat or sunlight. I'm going to transport you to the hospital now, where you can receive further treatment and care.

医生:不要触摸或抓挠水疱,这很重要,因为这样可能会导致水疱破裂并发生感染。烫伤部位要避免受热和晒到太阳。我现在要将您送往医院,在那里,您可以接受进一步治疗和护理。

**Patient:** OK, thank you for your help.

病人:好的,谢谢您的帮助。

**Doctor:** You're welcome. Please try to stay calm and relaxed. We'll get you to the hospital as soon as possible.

医生:不客气。请尽量保持冷静和放松。我们会尽快将您送到医院。

## Useful Expressions

Can you tell me how you got this burn?

您能告诉我您是怎么被烫伤的吗?

Where exactly is the burn located?

具体的烫伤部位在哪里?

On a scale of 1 to 10, with 10 being the worst, how would you rate your pain from the burn?

用 1 到 10 分来评估,10 分为最痛,您会给您的烫伤疼痛程度打几分？

Does the burn look like it blistered or peeled any skin?

烫伤部位有没有出现水疱或皮肤脱落？

I'm checking the appearance, size, and depth of the burn.

我来检查一下伤口的外观、大小和深度。

It looks like you have second-degree burns.

看起来像是Ⅱ度烫伤。

The top layers of skin are damaged.

表层皮肤已经受损。

We need to cool down the burns right away to prevent further damage.

我们需要尽快降温，以防止进一步的感染。

Don't touch or break any blisters, that could lead to infection. I'm going to clean the area and apply a sterile dressing.

不要触碰或刺破水疱，这样会导致感染。我给您清洁一下伤口，并敷上无菌敷料。

You should avoid exposing the burns to heat or sunlight.

烫伤部位要避免受热或晒到太阳。

## 3. Chemical Burn 化学性灼伤

## Conversation

**Patient, male, 23 years old, a chemistry student, accidentally spilled strong acid on his arm in the laboratory, resulting in a**

> 🔍 **Key Words and Phrases**
>
> **peel** [piːl] v. 脱落；adj. 去皮的
> **acid** [ˈæsɪd] n. 酸

chemical burn. **He immediately flushed the affected area with water and called for emergency medical services.**

病人,男性,23 岁,化学专业学生,在实验室中不慎将强酸洒到了手臂上,导致化学性灼伤。他立即用水冲洗受伤部位,并拨打了 120 急救电话。

**Doctor:** Hello, I'm the doctor responding to a chemical burn call. Can you tell me what happened?

医生:您好,我是受理化学性灼伤求助电话的医护人员。您能告诉我发生了什么事吗?

**Patient:** Hi, I'm a chemistry student and was working in the lab. I accidentally spilled some strong acid on my arm when I was handling a beaker.

病人:您好,我是一名化学专业的学生,在实验室里做实验,在处理一个烧杯时,我不小心将一些强酸溅到了手臂上。

**Doctor:** OK, what kind of acid was it?

医生:好的,是什么类型的酸?

**Patient:** It was 37% hydrochloric acid. I immediately rinsed my arm with water for 15 minutes after it spilled. But there is a nasty chemical burn on my forearm now.

病人: 是 37% 的盐酸。事后我立即用水冲洗了手臂 15 分钟。但现在我的前臂上有严重的化学性烧伤。

**Doctor:** You did the right

> **Key Words and Phrases**
>
> **beaker** [ˈbiːkə(r)] n. 烧杯,高脚杯
> **hydrochloric** [ˌhaɪdrəˈklɒrɪk] adj. 含氢和氯的
> **rinse** [rɪns] v. 漂洗
> **nasty** [ˈnɑːsti] adj. 造成很大伤害的

thing by flushing it. That can help prevent further burning. Let me take a look at your arm. Hmm yes, this is a severe chemical burn. It looks very red and inflamed. I'm going to wrap it with a sterile dressing. Are you feeling any pain or tingling?

**医生**：您冲洗伤口是对的，这有助于防止进一步烧伤。让我看看您的手臂。嗯，这确实是严重的化学性烧伤，看起来红肿严重，我要用无菌敷料把它包扎起来。您感觉疼痛或刺痛吗？

**Patient:** Yes, it is quite painful and my arm feels numb around the burn.

**病人**：是的，非常疼，而且我手臂的烧伤部位周围感觉麻。

**Doctor:** Alright, we need to get you to the hospital to properly treat this chemical burn. Burns like this can cause a lot of damage to the tissues and may require debridement. We'll transport you there right away and the doctor will be able to provide medication for the pain. Try to keep the arm elevated on the ride over. Let me know if you have any other questions.

**医生**：好的，我们需要把您送到医院，进行妥善处理。像这样的烧伤会对组织造成很大损害，可能需要进行清创手术。我们会立即把您送过去，医生可以为您提供止痛药物。在过去的路上，尽量保持手臂抬高。如果您还有其他问题，请告诉我。

**Patient:** OK, I really appreciate the help.

**病人**：好的，谢谢你们的帮助。

---

**🔍 Key Words and Phrases**

**inflamed** [ɪnˈfleɪmd] adj. 发炎的，红肿的

**tingling** [ˈtɪŋglɪŋ] n. 麻刺感

**debridement** [dɪˈbrɪdmənt] n. 清创术，扩创术（即清除伤口腐肉的手术）

## Useful Expressions

Can you tell me what type of chemical caused this burn?

您能告诉我是哪种化学物品引起的灼伤吗?

Where on your body did the chemical make contact?

您身体的哪个部位接触了化学物品?

Did you take any protective measures when the chemical spill occurred?

化学物品泼洒后,您采取了什么防护措施吗?

Is there still any chemicals remaining on the skin? We need to irrigate the area to flush out any remnants.

您的皮肤上还有化学物品残留吗? 我们需要冲洗该区域,清除残留物。

This looks like a second-degree burn with serious blistering and peeling of the skin layers.

有严重的水疱和皮肤脱落,看起来像是Ⅱ度烧伤。

Any burns to the eyes, nose or mouth?

眼睛、鼻子或嘴巴有没有灼伤?

I'm going to wrap the wound in a sterile dressing after irrigation. We'll get you to the emergency room for further treatment.

清洗后我会给您的伤口包上无菌敷料。我们要将您送去急诊进行进一步治疗。

> **🔍 Key Words and Phrases**
>
> **flush out** 把大量液体灌入……冲洗
>
> **remnant** ['remnənt] n. 残留物

# 4. Flame Burn 火焰烧伤

## Conversation

**Patient, female, 50 years old, was burned in a fire. She immediately called for emergency medical services.**

病人,女性,50 岁,在火灾中烧伤。她立即拨打了 120 急救电话。

**Doctor:** Hello ma'am, I'm the doctor. Can you tell me how did you get burnt?

医生:女士您好,我是急救医生。您能告诉我您是怎么被烧伤的吗?

**Patient:** There was a fire in my kitchen. I got burned on my face, arms and chest trying to escape.

病人:我家厨房着火了,在逃生的时候,我的脸、胳膊和胸部都被烧伤了。

**Doctor:** OK, those are definitely some serious burns. On a scale of 1 to 10, with 10 being the worst, how would you rate your pain?

医生:了解,这确实是非常严重的烧伤。用 1 到 10 分来评估,10 分为最痛,您会给您的疼痛程度打多少分?

**Patient:** The pain is severe, at least an 8 or 9.

病人:非常痛,至少是 8 或 9 分。

**Doctor:** Did you take any

> **🔍 Key Words and Phrases**
>
> **flame** [fleɪm] n. 火焰

first aid measures after getting burnt?

医生:烧伤后您有采取急救措施吗?

**Patient:** I have covered the injured areas with wet towels before you arrive.

病人:你们来之前,我用湿毛巾把伤口包住了。

**Doctor:** Alright, you did the right thing by covering the burns with wet towels. Let me check the affected area for signs of blistering or charring.

医生:您使用湿毛巾覆盖烧伤部位是正确的。让我检查一下烧伤区域,看看是否有水疱或被烧焦的迹象。

*The doctor examines the wounds.*

*医生检查了伤口。*

**Doctor:** There appears to be some blistering and charring of the skin, and it may be a second-degree burn.

医生:皮肤上出现了一些水疱,同时有被烧焦的迹象,可能是Ⅱ度烧伤。

**Patient:** Please help me.

病人:请帮帮我。

**Doctor:** Try to calm down. I am going to clean your wounds first. And then wrap some sterile dressings around the burnt areas. Let's get you onto the stretcher and into the ambulance.

医生:请尽量保持冷静。我现在要先清洁一下您的伤口,然后在烫伤的部位覆盖无菌敷料。让我们把您抬上担架,送到救护车上去吧。

*The patient is transferred*

> **🔍 Key Words and Phrases**
>
> **blister** [ˈblɪstər] v. 起疱
>
> **char** [tʃɑːr] v. 烧焦,炭化

*to the ambulance.*

*病人被送上救护车。*

**Doctor:** I'm concerned about the possibility of an <u>inhalation</u> injury if you were exposed to smoke or steam. Do you have difficulty breathing?

医生：如果接触了烟雾或蒸汽，我担心您可能有吸入性损伤。您觉得呼吸困难吗？

**Patient:** Yes, a little bit.

病人：有一点儿。

**Doctor:** We'll provide oxygen for you to help you breathe easier. We'll also get you some pain medications to relieve your pain.

医生：我们会给您供氧，让您呼吸得更顺畅些。我们还会为您提供一些止痛药以缓解疼痛。

**Patient:** Thank you.

病人：谢谢。

**Doctor:** We'll get you to the hospital right away where they can properly treat your burns. Try to take slow steady breaths. Let me know if the pain worsens or if you feel nauseous or faint on the way to the hospital.

医生：我们会立即将您送往医院，在那里他们能妥善处理您的烧伤。尽量缓慢平稳地呼吸。如果在去医院的路上疼痛加剧或感到恶心或头晕，请告知我。

**Patient:** OK, thank you.

病人：好的，谢谢。

> 🔍 **Key Words and Phrases**
>
> **inhalation** [ˌɪnhəˈleɪʃn] n. 吸入

## Useful Expressions

Can you tell me how did you get burnt?

您能告诉我您是如何被烧伤的吗?

Did you take any first aid measures after getting burnt?

烧伤后您有采取急救措施吗?

Let me check the affected area for signs of blistering or charring.

让我检查一下烧伤区域, 看看是否有水疱或被烧焦的迹象。

There appears to be some blistering and charring of the skin, and it may be a second-degree burn.

皮肤出现了一些水疱, 同时有被烧焦的迹象, 可能是Ⅱ度烧伤。

I am going to clean your wounds first. And then wrap some sterile dressings around the burnt areas.

我现在要先清洁一下您的伤口, 然后在烫伤的部位覆盖无菌敷料。

I'm concerned about the possibility of an inhalation injury if you were exposed to smoke or steam. Do you have difficulty breathing?

如果接触了烟雾或蒸汽, 我担心您可能有吸入性损伤。您觉得呼吸困难吗?

We'll provide oxygen for you to help you breathe easier.

我们会给您供氧让您呼吸得更顺畅些。

We'll get you some pain medications to relieve your pain.

我们会为您提供一些止痛药以缓解疼痛。

We need to get you to the hospital quickly so the doctors can properly clean and treat the wound.

我们需要尽快将您送往医院,这样医生才能对伤口进行适当清洁和处理。

Let me know if the pain worsens or if you feel nauseous or faint on the way to the hospital.

如果在去医院的路上疼痛加剧或感到恶心或头晕,请告知我。

# Section 5    Animal Bite (Sting) Injuries
# 动物咬(蜇)伤

## 1. Dog Bite 狗咬伤

### Conversation

**Patient, female, 6 years old, was bitten by a stray dog while playing in the park. Her parents immediately called for emergency medical services.**

患儿,女性,6 岁,在公园玩耍时被一只流浪狗咬伤,她的家长立即拨打了 120 急救电话。

**Doctor:** Hello, my name is Li Hua, and I'm a doctor. I understand that your daughter was bitten by a dog. Can you tell me more about

**Key Words and Phrases**

sting [stɪŋ] n. 蜇伤处
stray [streɪ] adj.（常指宠物）走失的

what happened?

医生：您好，我叫李华，是一名急救医生。我了解到您的女儿被狗咬了，可以把详细情况再跟我说一下吗？

**Patient's family member:** Of course. My daughter was playing in the park, and suddenly a dog came <u>out of nowhere</u> and bit her on her right lower leg. The wound looked quite deep, and there was a lot of blood. She feels very painful right now.

病人家属：当然。我女儿在公园里玩，突然不知道从哪里冒出来一只狗，咬了她的右小腿。伤口看起来很深，流了很多血。她觉得非常痛。

**Doctor:** Let me take a look at her wound. Can you please help me remove her shoe and sock so I can see the bite?

医生：让我来检查一下她的伤口。您可以帮我脱掉她的鞋和袜子，让我看看伤口吗？

**Patient's family member:** Sure, here you go.

病人家属：当然，您看。

**Doctor:** Thank you. The wound looks quite deep, and it's bleeding heavily. We need to clean it up and <u>bandage</u> it to prevent further infection.

医生：谢谢。伤口看起来很深，流了很多血。我们需要清理伤口并包扎好，避免进一步感染。

**Patient's family member:** OK, what should we do?

病人家属：好的，我们应该怎么做？

> **🔍 Key Words and Phrases**
>
> **out of nowhere** 突然冒出来
>
> **bandage** [ˈbændɪdʒ] v. 用绷带包扎

**Doctor:** First, we will apply pressure to the wound to stop the bleeding. It might hurt a little. After that, we need to squeeze the blood out from the wound so that we can clear the toxin. Then, we will clean the wound by using saline solution to prevent infection. Finally, we'll wrap the wound with sterile dressings.

医生：首先，需要按压伤口止血，可能会有点儿疼。然后，需要挤出伤口污血，这样才能清除毒素。接着，用盐水清洗伤口，以防止感染。最后，用无菌敷料包扎好伤口。

**Patient's family member:** OK, please go ahead.

病人家属：好的，请开始吧。

*The doctor and the nurse perform a series of emergency cares.*

急救人员进行了一系列急救护理。

**Doctor:** We've controlled the bleeding for now. But I'm concerned about infection so we'll get her to the hospital quickly to clean the wound properly. She may need some stitches and antibiotics. Was the dog a stray?

医生：我们暂时止住了血。但是我担心会感染，所以我们会尽快把她送到医院，妥善地清创。她可能需要缝针和注射抗生素。那条狗是流浪狗吗？

**Patient's family member:** Yes, I believe so. I'm not sure if it had a rabies vaccine.

> **🔍 Key Words and Phrases**
>
> **squeeze** [skwiːz] v. 挤压
>
> **toxin** [ˈtɒksɪn] n. 毒素
>
> **saline** [ˈseɪlaɪn] adj. 含盐的
>
> **solution** [səˈluːʃn] n. 溶解，解决办法，答案
>
> **stitch** [stɪtʃ] n. (缝合伤口的) 缝针
>
> **rabies vaccine** 狂犬病疫苗

**病人家属**：应该是的，我不确定它是否接种了狂犬病疫苗。

**Doctor:** OK, the doctor in the hospital may decide to give her the rabies vaccine as a precaution. Let's get her into the ambulance and to the hospital.

**医生**：好的，为了以防万一，医院里的医生可能会为她注射狂犬病疫苗。让我们把她送上救护车，送往医院。

**Patient's family member:** Alright, thank you for your help.

**病人家属**：好的，感谢你们的帮助。

## Useful Expressions

What kind of dog bit you? Was it a large breed or small breed?

您是被哪种狗咬的，是大型犬还是小型犬？

Did the dog break the skin or was it just a scratch?

狗咬破了皮肤，还是只是轻微刮伤？

Can you tell me where the bite occurred on the body?

您能告诉我狗咬在哪个部位了吗？

Have you noticed any signs of infection, such as redness, swelling, or discharge?

有没有出现感染的迹象？比如红肿或有分泌物。

Have you had a <u>tetanus</u> shot?

您是否接种过破伤风疫苗？

Do you know the owner of the dog?

您能告诉我狗咬在哪个部位了吗？

> 🔍 **Key Words and Phrases**
>
> **tetanus** ['tetənəs] n. 破伤风

您知道狗的主人是谁吗？

Was the dog vaccinated against rabies?

这只狗是否注射了狂犬病疫苗？

We need to stop the bleeding by applying pressure to the wound.

我们需要通过按压伤口来止血。

We will squeeze the blood out from the wound so that the toxin can be sucked out.

我们将挤出伤口污血，这样才能排出毒素。

We'll clean the wound with saline solution to prevent any infection.

我们将用盐水清洗伤口，以防止感染。

We'll cover the wound with a sterile dressing and bandage it up.

我们会用无菌敷料覆盖伤口并包扎好。

## 2. Spider Bite 蜘蛛咬伤

## Conversation

**Patient, male, 35 years old, was bitten by a spider on his left hand while camping outdoors. The patient called for emergency medical services.**

病人，男性，35 岁，在郊外露营时被蜘蛛咬伤了左手，该病人拨打了 120 急救电话。

**Doctor:** Sir, I'm the doctor. Can you tell me how did you

🔍 **Key Words and Phrases**

**spider** [ˈspaɪdə(r)] n. 蜘蛛

get the bite?

医生：先生，我是医护人员。您能告诉我您是怎么被咬伤的吗？

**Patient:** I was camping and a spider bit me on my left hand. It really hurts and now my hand is swollen.

病人：在露营时，一只蜘蛛咬了我的左手，真的很痛，现在我的手肿了。

**Doctor:** OK, spider bites can be painful. Let me take a look at your hand. Does it feel numb or tingling?

医生：好的，蜘蛛咬伤是很痛的。让我看看您的手，有麻木或刺痛感吗？

**Patient:** Yes, it feels numb and is tingling a lot.

病人：是的，我感觉我的手发麻，而且非常刺痛。

**Doctor:** Alright, I'm going to wrap a bandage to <u>immobilize</u> your hand. This should help slow the <u>venom</u> from spreading. Then I will clean the wound with a weak <u>acidic</u> solution.

医生：好的，我要将您的手包扎固定住。这应该有助于减缓毒液的扩散。然后我会用弱酸性溶液清洗一下您的伤口。

**Patient:** Will I be OK? Do I need any medications?

病人：我会没事的吧，我需不需要吃什么药？

**Doctor:** You will be fine. I will give you some pain relief

---

🔍 **Key Words and Phrases**

**immobilize** [ɪˈməʊbəlaɪz] v. 使不动

**venom** [ˈvenəm] n. (某些蛇、蝎子等分泌的)毒液

**acidic** [əˈsɪdɪk] adj. <化>酸的

to help you feel better. And I'll monitor your vital signs closely. Let me know if you have trouble breathing or the swelling spreads.

医生：您会没事的。我会为您提供一些止痛药帮您缓解疼痛。同时我会密切监测您的生命体征。如果您觉得呼吸困难或肿胀扩散了就告诉我。

**Patient:** OK, thank you.

病人：好的，谢谢。

**Doctor:** No problem, sir. We're going to get you to the hospital. Spider bites can sometimes cause more severe reactions, so the emergency room doctor will want to monitor you for a few hours and give you antibiotics as a precaution.

医生：不客气，先生。我们要把您送到医院。蜘蛛咬伤有时会引起严重的反应，所以急诊医生会对您进行几个小时的监测，并预防性给予抗生素。

**Patient:** That would be great, thank you.

病人：那太好了，谢谢你们。

## Useful Expressions

Can you tell me how did you get the bite?

您能告诉我您是怎么被咬的吗？

Does the wound feel numb or tingling?

有感觉伤口麻木或刺痛吗？

I'm going to wrap a bandage to immobilize your hand. This should help slow the venom from spreading.

我要将您的手包扎固定住。这应该有助于减缓毒液的扩散。

I will clean the wound with a weak acidic solution.

我会用弱酸性溶液清洗一下您的伤口。

I will give you some pain relief to help you feel better.

我会为您提供一些止痛药帮您缓解疼痛。

Let me know if you have trouble breathing or the swelling spreads.

如果您觉得呼吸困难或肿胀扩散了就告诉我。

Spider bites can sometimes cause more severe reactions.

蜘蛛咬伤有时会引起严重的反应。

# 3. Snake Bite 蛇咬伤

## Conversation

**Patient, female, 22 years old, was bitten by a snake while hiking in the wilderness. Her friend called for emergency medical services.**

病人，女性，22 岁，在野外徒步时，被蛇咬伤，她的朋友拨打了 120 急救电话。

**Doctor:** Hello, my name is Li Hua, and I'm a paramedic. I understand that you were bitten by a snake. Can you tell me how did you get the bite?

医生：您好，我是李华，是一名急救医生。我了解到您被蛇咬伤了，您能告诉我您是怎么被咬伤的吗？

**Patient:** Yes, I was hiking with some friends. And I

accidentally stepped on something soft. It turned out to be a snake. The snake bit me on my ankle, and now my ankle is swollen and very painful.

**病人:**好的。我当时正和几个朋友在徒步,不小心踩到了一个软软的东西,结果是一条蛇。它咬了我的脚踝,我的脚踝现在肿了,而且很痛。

**Doctor:** Can you describe the type of the snake?

**医生:**您能描述一下那条蛇长什么样吗?

**Patient:** It has black stripes, and the color seems to be brownish yellow.

**病人:**它有黑色的条纹,好像是棕黄色的。

*The doctor examines the wound.*

*医生检查伤口。*

**Doctor:** This looks like a bite from a rattlesnake. I can see some swelling and redness around the wound. This is a serious situation, and we need to act fast.

**医生:**这看起来像是响尾蛇造成的咬伤。我可以看到伤口周围有些肿胀和发红。这比较严重,我们需要迅速行动。

**Patient:** What should we do?

**病人:**应该怎么办呢?

**Doctor:** First, we need to clean the wound with soap water

---

🔍 **Key Words and Phrases**

**turn out to be** 结果是,原来是

**stripe** [ˈstraɪp] n. 条纹

**rattlesnake** [ˈrætlsneɪk] n. 响尾蛇

to prevent any infection. After that, we'll apply a compression bandage to the bite to slow down the spread of venom throughout your body.

医生：首先，我们需要用肥皂水清洗伤口以防止感染。之后，我们会在咬伤处绑上压力绷带，减缓毒液在您身体中扩散。

**Patient:** Alright.

病人：好的。

**Doctor:** Keep your leg still. I'm giving you an antivenom injection as well as some oral medications to counteract the venom.

医生：不要动您的腿。我会为您注射抗毒血清并提供一些口服药物，以中和毒液。

**Patient:** Oh, thank you! Will I be OK though?

病人：好的，谢谢！我会没事的吧？

**Doctor:** We need to monitor your condition closely to ensure that the venom doesn't cause any severe reactions. Can you tell me if you feel any dizziness, nausea, or shortness of breath?

医生：我们还需要密切监测您的状况，确保毒液不会引起严重反应。请问您是否感到头晕、恶心或呼吸困难？

**Patient:** No, I don't feel any of those symptoms right now.

病人：没有，这些症状都没有。

**Doctor:** Alright, that's a good sign. We'll keep monitoring you and transport you to the hospital for further treatment.

---

🔍 **Key Words and Phrases**

**compression bandage** < 医 > 压迫绷带

**counteract** [ˌkaʊntərˈækt] v. 抵制

**医生**：那就好，这是个好迹象。我们会继续监测您的情况，并将您转运到医院，进行进一步治疗。

**Patient:** Alright, thank you for your help.

**病人**：好的，谢谢你们的帮忙。

## Useful Expressions

Can you tell me how did you get the bite?

您能告诉我您是怎么被咬的吗？

Can you describe the type of the snake?

您能描述一下那条蛇长什么样吗？

I can see some swelling and redness around the wound.

我可以看到伤口周围有些肿胀和发红。

This is a serious situation, and we need to act fast.

这比较严重，我们需要迅速行动。

We need to clean the wound with soap water to prevent any infection.

我们需要用肥皂水清洗伤口以防止感染。

We'll apply a compression bandage to the bite to slow down the spread of venom throughout your body.

我们会在咬伤处绑上压力绷带，减缓毒液在您身体中扩散。

I'm giving you an antivenom injection as well as some oral medications to counteract the venom.

我会为您注射抗毒血清并提供一些口服药物，以中和毒液。

Can you tell me if you feel any dizziness, nausea, or shortness of breath?

请问您是否感到头晕、恶心或呼吸困难？

We'll keep monitoring you and transport you to the hospital for further treatment.

我们会继续监测您的情况,并将您转运到医院,进行进一步治疗。

# Unit 5

## Common Acute Poisonings
## 常见急性中毒

### Section 1　Food Poisoning
### 食物中毒

#### Conversation

Patient, female, 23 years old, began to experience <u>abdominal</u> pain, vomiting, and diarrhea after lunch. The patient called for emergency medical services.

病人，女性，23 岁，午饭后开始出现腹痛、呕吐和腹泻症状。病人拨打了 120 急救电话。

**Doctor:** Hello, I'm a doctor from 120 Emergency. What seems to be the problem?

医生：您好！我是 120 急救中心的医生。请问发生了什么事？

**Patient:** Hi! I started

🔍 **Key Words and Phrases**

**food poisoning** 食物中毒
**abdominal** [æbˈdɒmɪnl] adj. 腹部的

feeling abdominal pain, nauseous and then vomiting and diarrhea after I had lunch.

病人：您好！吃过午饭后，我开始感到肚子疼、恶心，然后开始呕吐、腹泻。

**Doctor:** How long have you been experiencing these symptoms?

医生：您的症状持续多长时间了？

**Patient:** It started about an hour ago and it's getting worse.

病人：大概是一个小时前开始的，越来越糟糕。

**Doctor:** How many times have you vomited and had diarrhea?

医生：您呕吐和腹泻了大概多少次？

**Patient:** At least 4 or 5 times each.

病人：至少四五次。

**Doctor:** Any blood or mucus in the stool?

医生：排泄物中有血丝或黏液吗？

**Patient:** Yes, there were some blood and mucus.

病人：是的，有一些血丝和黏液。

**Doctor:** Have you had any illnesses recently or taken any new medications?

医生：您最近有生病或服用新药吗？

**Patient:** No.

病人：没有。

**Doctor:** Have you eaten anything unusual or gone to any new places recently?

医生：您最近吃过什么不常吃的食物或去过什么新

🔍 **Key Words and Phrases**

**stool** [stu:l] n. 大便，凳子，高脚凳

地方吗?

**Patient:** Actually, I did try a new restaurant for lunch today. Maybe it was something I ate there?

**病人:**事实上,我今天去了一家新的餐馆吃午饭。难道是吃了那里的什么东西导致的?

**Doctor:** Have any other family members or friends who ate the same foods also become ill?

**医生:**有其他家人或者朋友吃了同样的食物后也不舒服吗?

**Patient:** I only had lunch by myself.

**病人:**我是自己一个人去吃的午饭。

**Doctor:** Based on your symptoms, it sounds like you may have food poisoning. We need to get you to the hospital to be evaluated and treated further. Now I'll start intravenous infusion and give you some medications to help with the nausea, vomiting and diarrhea. And I'll collect some vomits for further diagnosis and treatment in hospital.

**医生:**根据您的症状判断,您可能是食物中毒了。我们需要把您送到医院,进行进一步检查和治疗。现在,我将为您静脉输液并给您服用一些药物,以缓解恶心、呕吐和腹泻症状。并且,我会收集一些呕吐物,帮助医院进一步诊断和治疗。

**Patient:** OK. Thank you.

**病人:**好的。谢谢!

## Useful Expressions

Have you experienced any nausea or vomiting?

您是否有恶心或呕吐?

Have you had any diarrhea or abdominal pain?

您是否有腹泻或腹痛的症状?

How long have you been experiencing these symptoms?

您的症状持续多长时间了?

How many times have you vomited and had diarrhea?

您呕吐和腹泻了多少次?

Any blood or mucus in the stool?

排泄物中有血丝或黏液吗?

Have you had any recent illnesses or taken any new medications?

您最近有生病或服用新药吗?

Have you eaten anything unusual or eaten at a new restaurant recently?

您最近吃过不常吃的东西或去过新的餐厅吗?

Have you traveled recently or been in contact with anyone who has been ill?

您最近有旅行或接触过病人吗?

Have any other family members or friends who ate the same foods also become ill?

有家人或者朋友吃了同样的食物后也不舒服吗?

It's possible that you have food poisoning.

您可能是食物中毒。

I'm going to give you an anti-nausea medication to help with the vomiting and an oral rehydration solution to prevent dehydration.

我会给您服用止呕药以缓

> **Key Words and Phrases**
>
> oral rehydration solution 口服补盐液

解呕吐,并服用口服补液盐以防止脱水。

I'll collect some vomits for further diagnosis and treatment in hospital

我会收集一些呕吐物,帮助医院进一步诊断和治疗。

# Section 2　Drug Poisoning
# 药物中毒

## Conversation

**Patient, female, 13 years old, accidentally took an <u>overdose</u> of <u>sedatives</u>, resulting in unconsciousness and difficulty breathing. Her family member immediately called for emergency medical services.**

病人,女性,13 岁,误食过量镇静剂,出现昏迷和呼吸困难,家属立即拨打了 120 急救电话。

**Doctor:** Hello, I'm an EMT. Can you tell me exactly what happened?

医生:您好,我是急救医生。您能告诉我到底发生了什么事情吗?

**Patient's family member:** It's my daughter, she has accidentally taken too many of her <u>sleeping pills</u>. I think she has overdosed. She's unconscious and not breathing well.

> **🔍 Key Words and Phrases**
>
> **overdose** [ˈəʊvədəʊs] n. 服药过量
>
> **sedative** [ˈsedətɪv] n. 镇静药,镇静剂
>
> **sleeping pill** 安眠药片

**病人家属**：是我女儿，她不小心吃了太多安眠药，我觉得她服药过量了。她昏迷了并且呼吸困难。

**Doctor:** OK, try to stay calm. How old is your daughter?

**医生**：好的，请尽量保持冷静。您女儿多大年纪？

**Patient's family member:** She's 13 years old.

**病人家属**：她13岁。

**Doctor:** Alright, we're going to take good care of her. Can you tell me what kind of drug the patient may have taken?

**医生**：好的，我们会好好照顾她的。请问病人可能吃了什么药？

**Patient's family member:** It was clonazepam, her sleep medication. The bottle is still open on the table.

**病人家属**：是氯硝西泮，她的安眠药。药瓶还开着，在桌子上。

**Doctor:** When did she take the drugs?

**医生**：她什么时候服用的药物？

**Patient's family member:** About half an hour ago.

**病人家属**：大概半小时前。

**Doctor:** Did the patient have any nausea, vomiting, confusion, seizure activity?

**医生**：病人有恶心、呕吐、意识混乱、抽搐等症状吗？

**Patient's family member:** No, when I found her, she has lost her consciousness.

**病人家属**：没有，我看到她的时候，她已经失去意识了。

**Doctor:** OK, we'll need to

> **🔍 Key Words and Phrases**
>
> **clonazepam** [kləʊˈnəzpæm]
> n. 氯硝西泮

know the package and how many pills are missing to determine the amount she took. But first we need to make sure she's stable and breathing. Now my partner is going to assess her condition and provide oxygen.

医生：好的，我们需要知道剂量和药瓶里少了多少药，以确定她吃了多少。不过首先我们需要确保她情况稳定并且能正常呼吸。现在，我的搭档会开始评估她的情况，并给她供氧。

*The nurse begins helping assess the patient and provide emergency medical care.*

*护士开始评估病人并提供医疗救助。*

**Doctor:** Ma'am, we're going to take your daughter to the hospital right away to have gastric lavage and other treatment for the overdose. You can ride with us in the ambulance.

医生：女士，我们要立即将您女儿送到医院，为她进行洗胃及其他的药物过量治疗。您可以乘坐救护车和我们一起去。

**Patient's family member:** Thank you so much. Please do everything you can to help her.

病人家属：太谢谢你们了。请尽一切可能救救她。

**Doctor:** We will. Don't worry.

医生：我们会的。不用担心。

## Useful Expressions

Can you tell me what kind of drug the patient may have

🔍 **Key Words and Phrases**

**gastric lavage** 洗胃

taken?

请问病人可能吃了什么药？

When did he / she take the medications / drugs?

他 / 她是什么时候服用的药物？

How much did he / she take?

他 / 她服用了多少剂量？

Did the patient have any nausea, vomiting, confusion, seizure activity?

病人有恶心、呕吐、意识混乱、抽搐等症状吗？

Does the patient have any history of drug abuse or addiction?

病人是否有药物滥用史或药物成瘾史？

Let's get some oxygen on and monitor his / her breathing closely.

我们要进行供氧治疗，并密切监测他 / 她的呼吸。

I'm going to start an intravenous injection and give him / her some medications to help reverse the overdose effects.

我将进行静脉注射，给予他 / 她一些药物以帮助治疗药物过量。

We need to transport him to the hospital right away for further monitoring and treatment.

我们需要立即将他转运到医院，进行进一步监测和治疗。

Bring the pill bottles and anything involved so we can show doctors.

把药瓶和相关的东西都带上，以便给医生看。

# Section 3　Acute Carbon Monoxide Poisoning 急性一氧化碳中毒

## Conversation

**Patient, male, 28 years old, suddenly collapsed and lost consciousness while taking a shower at home. His family member immediately called for emergency medical services.**

病人,男性,28 岁,在家中洗澡时,突然倒地昏迷,家属发现后拨打了 120 急救电话。

**Doctor:** Hi, I'm Li Hua, a paramedic. Are you a family member of the patient?

**医生:**您好,我叫李华,是急救医生。您是病人的家属吗?

**Patient's family member:** Yes, I'm his wife. Is my husband going to be OK?

**病人家属:**是的,我是他的妻子。我的丈夫没事吧?

**Doctor:** We're doing everything we can to help your husband. Can you tell me what happened before he collapsed?

**医生:**我们会尽力帮助您的丈夫。请问在他晕倒之前发生了什么事?

**Patient's family member:** He was taking a shower using the gas water heater at home and suddenly collapsed. He's unconscious now and not waking up.

> ### 🔍 Key Words and Phrases
>
> **carbon monoxide** 一氧化碳
> **collapse** [kəˈlæps] v. 倒下
> **water heater** 热水器

**病人家属**：他当时在家里用燃气热水器洗澡，突然就晕倒了。他现在没有意识，也没有醒过来。

**Doctor:** Did you smell any gas before or after he collapsed?

医生：他晕倒之前您有闻到煤气的味道吗?

**Patient's family member:** Yes, I think I smelled some gas.

病人家属：有，我闻到了煤气的味道。

**Doctor:** Your husband may have been using a gas water heater for a long time, but there was no <u>ventilation</u>, resulting in carbon monoxide poisoning. We will do our best to save him. Before we start treatment, could you please open the windows to let the air <u>circulate</u>?

医生：您的丈夫可能是用燃气热水器洗澡，但是长时间没有通风，导致一氧化碳中毒。我们会尽力救治他。在开始之前，请您开窗让空气流通起来。

**Patient's family member:** OK, I'll go open the windows right away.

病人家属：好的，我现在就去开窗。

**Doctor:** Thank you. Can you tell me what symptoms your husband has been experiencing?

医生：谢谢。您能描述一下您丈夫的症状吗?

**Patient's family member:** He's been confused, breathing rapidly, and his lips and face are cherry red. I'm very worried about him.

病人家属：他意识模糊，呼吸急促，嘴巴和面部都呈樱桃红色，我很担心他。

> **Key Words and Phrases**
>
> **ventilation** [ˌventɪˈleɪʃən] n. 空气流通
> **circulate** [ˈsɜːkjəleɪt] v. 循环

**Doctor:** It sounds like carbon monoxide poisoning. I'll take his vital signs.

医生：听起来是一氧化碳中毒。我要测量一下他的生命体征。

*After examining the patient.*

*检查之后。*

**Doctor:** Luckily, he still has heartbeat, but his pulse is too weak. We need to move him to the ambulance now. Can you tell me if he has any allergies or medical conditions we should know about?

医生：很幸运，他还有心跳，但是脉搏非常弱。我们现在需要马上将他转移到救护车上。请问他有过敏史或疾病史吗？

**Patient's family member:** No.

病人家属：没有。

*The patient is transferred to the ambulance.*

*病人被转移到救护车上。*

**Doctor:** Now we will put an oxygen mask on him to help him breathe more easily, and my partner will get some intravenous injection fluids ready. And we will monitor him closely through the electrocardiogram all the way to the hospital. The doctors will take good care of him.

医生：我们现在给他戴上氧气面罩，让他呼吸得更顺畅一些，我的搭档也会对他进行静脉输液。去医院的路上，我们会通过心电监护对他进行密切监测，医院的医生会照顾好他的。

**Patient's family member:** OK, thank you very much. Please help him.

病人家属：好的，非常感谢。请一定要救救他。

## Useful Expressions

Has the patient been exposed to any potential sources of carbon monoxide, such as a faulty furnace or gas water heater?

病人是否接触了一氧化碳的潜在来源？比如有故障的炉子或燃气热水器。

Is the patient conscious and responsive or unconscious?

病人是否有意识、有反应？

Does the patient have a headache, dizziness, nausea, vomiting, or loss of consciousness?

病人是否头痛、头晕、恶心、呕吐或丧失意识？

Does the patient have a history of respiratory or heart problems?

病人是否有呼吸系统疾病或心脏病史？

The patient's lips and fingernails look red.

病人的嘴唇和指甲看起来发红。

It's possible that the patient has acute carbon monoxide poisoning.

病人可能是急性一氧化碳中毒。

Where is the exposure source? Does anyone else feel sick?

暴露源在哪里，其他人是否也感到不适？

We need to ventilate the area and get everyone to fresh air immediately.

我们要立即通风，并将所有人都撤离到空气清新的地方去。

> **Key Words and Phrases**
>
> furnace ['fɜːnɪs] n. 熔炉

# Section 4    Pesticide Poisoning
# 农药中毒

## Conversation

Patient, male, 53 years old, experienced discomfort after spraying <u>insecticides</u> in his own garden. His family member immediately called for emergency medical services.

病人,男性,53 岁,在自家花园喷洒杀虫药后,出现了不适,他的家属立即拨打了 120 急救电话。

**Doctor:** Sir, can you tell me what happened?

医生:先生,您能告诉我发生了什么事吗?

**Patient:** I was spraying insecticides in my garden and suddenly started feeling unwell. I have a bad headache, feel dizzy and nauseous. I've been vomiting and have tears in my eyes too.

病人:我在花园里喷杀虫剂,突然感觉不适。我头疼得厉害,感到眩晕和恶心,还有呕吐和流泪的症状。

**Doctor:** I see. These symptoms are very likely to be pesticide poisoning. Let me do a quick check of your vital signs first.

医生:这些症状很可能是农药中毒导致的。我先为您做一个快速检查,看看您的生命体征。

*Doing examination.*

*进行检查。*

**Doctor:** Your blood pressure is slightly high, but other vital signs are generally normal. Please tell me, what kind of pesticide did you spray? And about how much did you spray?

医生：您的血压略高，但其他生命体征总体正常。请告诉我您喷洒的是什么农药，大概喷洒了多少？

Patient: I'm not very clear about the brand of pesticide. It seems to be some kind of insecticide. I sprayed about half a bottle of it. This is the bottle.

病人：我不太清楚是什么品牌的农药，好像是杀虫剂之类的。我大概喷洒了半瓶的量，这是它的瓶子。

Doctor: Can you tell me how long ago you sprayed them?

医生：您是多久之前进行喷洒的？

Patient: It was about an hour ago.

病人：大概一个小时前。

Doctor: Alright, we need to get you to the hospital as soon as possible for decontamination and further treatment. Please remove the clothing, shoes, and socks that have been contaminated with the toxic substance. Have you washed your hands thoroughly yet?

医生：好的，我们需要尽快把您送到医院进行排毒和进一步治疗。请换掉您的衣服、鞋子和袜子，它们都被污染了。您洗干净双手了吗？

Patient: No, not yet.

### 🔍 Key Words and Phrases

decontamination [ˌdiːkənˌtæmɪˈneɪʃn] n. 去污

contaminate [kənˈtæmɪneɪt] v. 污染

substance [ˈsʌbstəns] n. 物质

thoroughly [ˈθʌrəli] adv. 彻底地，认真仔细地，完全地

**病人：**还没有。

**Doctor:** OK, let's get you to wash your hands and face right now with soap and water.

**医生：**好的，我们现在协助您用肥皂水彻底清洗双手和脸部。

*The nurse assists the patient to do the washing.*

*护士帮助病人进行清洗。*

**Doctor:** How are you feeling now? Any difficulty breathing?

**医生：**您现在感觉怎么样，呼吸困难吗？

**Patient:** The nausea and headache are getting worse. But no trouble breathing so far.

**病人：**恶心和头痛还在加重，但是呼吸没有什么问题。

**Doctor:** That's good. I'm giving you an antiemetic to reduce the nausea and vomiting. My partner will provide oxygen for you, and get some intravenous injection fluids ready. And we will monitor you closely through the electrocardiogram all the way to the hospital. The doctors there will give you further treatments

**医生：**那就好。我给您服用一些止吐剂，以帮助您减轻恶心和呕吐。我的搭档会为您供氧和静脉输液。在去医院的路上，我们会通过心电监护密切监测您的情况，医院的医生会为您提供进一步治疗。

**Patient:** OK, thank you so much.

**病人：**好的，非常感谢。

**Doctor:** You're welcome.

**医生：**不客气。

## Useful Expressions

Has the patient been exposed to any pesticides or <u>chemicals</u> recently?

病人最近是否接触过农药或化学物质？

Is there any smell of chemicals in the area?

该区域是否有化学物质的气味？

Has the patient experienced any symptoms of pesticide poisoning, such as headache, dizziness, or nausea?

病人是否有农药中毒的症状？比如头痛、眩晕或恶心。

Is the patient conscious and responsive or unconscious?

病人是否有意识、有反应？

Does the patient have any respiratory or cardiac symptoms, such as difficulty breathing or chest pain?

病人是否有呼吸道或心脏症状？比如呼吸困难或胸痛。

What kind of pesticide did the patient spray? How much did the patient spray?

病人喷洒的是什么农药，喷洒了多少？

How long ago did the patient spray the pesticide?

病人是多久前喷洒农药的？

It's possible that the patient has pesticide poisoning.

病人可能是农药中毒。

The patient has some constricted pupils and labored breathing—signs of pesticide poisoning.

病人瞳孔缩小、呼吸困难——这些都是农药中毒的

> 🔍 **Key Words and Phrases**
>
> **chemical** [ˈkemɪkəl] n. 化学药品

体征。

Let's get the patient decontaminated by removing any contaminated clothes.

让我们帮病人清除毒物,脱掉被污染的衣服。

Let's assist the patient to wash his / her hands and face with soap and water.

让我们用肥皂水帮病人清洗他 / 她的手部和脸部。

We need to get him to the hospital for observation and blood examination.

我们需要送他去医院进行观察和血液检查。

Bring the pesticide <u>containers</u> or a sample of what was used.

带上农药容器或所使用农药的样本。

# Section 5   Alcoholism
# 酒精中毒

## Conversation

**Patient, male, 25 years old, drank a large amount of <u>alcohol</u> and developed symptoms such as shortness of breath, rapid heartbeat, confusion, and vomiting. His friend immediately called for emergency medical services.**

病人,男性,25 岁,喝了大量的酒,出现呼吸急促、心跳加速、意识模糊、呕吐等症状,他的朋友立即拨打了 120 急救电话。

> 🔍 **Key Words and Phrases**
>
> **container** [kənˈteɪmə] n. 容器
>
> **alcohol** [ˈælkəhɒl] n. 酒

**Doctor:** Hi, I'm a paramedic. What's wrong with your friend?

医生：您好，我是急救医生。您的朋友怎么了?

**Patient's friend:** He drank too much tonight and now he's experiencing some terrible symptoms.

病人朋友：我朋友今晚喝了太多酒了，现在出现了很多糟糕的症状。

**Doctor:** What symptoms has he been experiencing?

医生：他都出现了哪些症状?

**Patient's friend:** He's having difficulty breathing, and his heart rate is fast. He seems to be confused and has vomited a few times.

病人朋友：他呼吸困难，心跳很快，似乎神志不清，而且呕吐了好几次。

**Doctor:** OK, we'll take a look at him. Can you tell me his name and age?

医生：好的，我们来看看他。您能告知我他的姓名和年龄吗?

**Patient's friend:** His name is Jason, and he's 25 years old.

病人朋友：他叫贾森，今年 25 岁。

*The doctor examines the patient.*

*医生检查病人。*

**Doctor:** Jason, can you tell me what happened? How much did you drink?

医生：贾森，您能告诉我发生了什么事吗，您喝了多少酒?

**Patient:** *(mumbling incoherently)* …

---

🔍 **Key Words and Phrases**

**incoherently** [ˌɪnkəʊˈhɪərəntlɪ] adv. 语无伦次地

病人:(含糊不清地说)……

**Doctor:** His symptoms indicate alcohol poisoning. Can you tell me how much did he drink?

医生:他的症状看起来像是酒精中毒。您能告诉我他喝了多少酒吗?

**Patient's friend:** Yes, he was drinking some beer and hard liquor. But I'm not really sure how much he drank exactly.

病人朋友:他喝了一些啤酒和烈酒,但是我不太清楚他具体喝了多少。

**Doctor:** Did he take any medications before drinking, such as cephalosporin antibiotics?

医生:他喝酒前有没有服用什么药物? 比如头孢类药物。

**Patient's friend:** As far as I know, probably not.

病人朋友:据我所知,应该没有。

**Doctor:** Alright, let's make sure his airway is clear and he can breathe easily. We should turn his head to the side to prevent chocking by his vomits. And we need to get him on a monitor and start an intravenous injection to give him some fluids. His heartbeat is very fast and irregular, which can be dangerous.

医生:好的,我们要确保他的呼吸道通畅,能够顺畅呼吸,将他的头转向一侧,防止他被呕吐物噎住。同时,我们需要对他进行监护并开始静脉输液。他的心跳非常快且不规律,这会很危险。

**Patient's friend:** Will he be alright?

病人朋友:他会没事吧?

**Doctor:** These types of episodes can be very serious and even life-threatening. But if we can rehydrate him and manage his vitals, he should stabilize and recover fully.

医生:这些症状可能非常严重,甚至会威胁生命。但是如果我们能够给他补水,控制好他的各项生命体征,他的病情应该会稳定下来并且完全恢复。

**Patient's friend:** OK, please do everything you can to help him.

病人朋友:好的,请一定要救救他。

**Doctor:** Of course. We're going to take good care of your friend.

医生:当然。我们会照顾好您的朋友。

## Useful Expressions

What symptoms has the patient been experiencing?

病人都出现了哪些症状?

Can you tell me the patient's name and age?

您能告知我病人的姓名和年龄吗?

How much did the patient drink?

病人喝了多少酒?

Did the patient take any medications before drinking, such as cephalosporin antibiotics?

病人喝酒前有没有服用什么药物?比如头孢类药物。

It's possible that the patient has alcohol poisoning.

病人很有可能是酒精中毒。

Let's make sure the patient's airway is clear and he / she can breathe easily.

我们要确保病人的呼吸道通畅，能够顺畅呼吸。

We should turn the patient's head to the side to prevent chocking by his / her vomits.

我们应该将病人的头转向一侧，防止他 / 她被呕吐物噎住。

We need to get the patient on a monitor and start an intravenous injection to give him / her some fluids.

我们需要对病人进行监护，并开始进行静脉输液。

His / her heartbeat is very fast and irregular, which can be dangerous.

他 / 她的心跳非常快且不规律，这会很危险。

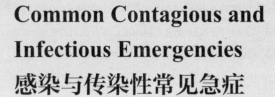

# Unit 6

## Common Contagious and Infectious Emergencies
## 感染与传染性常见急症

### Section 1　Measles
### 麻疹

## Conversation

Patient, male, 2 years old, developed a rash that covers his entire body. His family member called for emergency medical services.

患儿,男性,2 岁,全身出现皮疹,家属拨打了 120 急救电话。

**Doctor:** Hi, I'm a doctor from 120 Emergency. What seems to be the problem?

> **🔍 Key Words and Phrases**
>
> **contagious** [kənˈteɪdʒəs] adj.(病)感染性的
> **infectious** [ɪnˈfekʃəs] adj. 传染的
> **measles** [ˈmiːzlz] n. < 医 > 麻疹,< 兽 >(牛,猪的)囊虫病

医生：您好，我是 120 急救医生。请问发生了什么事？

**Patient's family member:** It's my son. He has been sick for several days. He developed a high fever, cough, runny nose and his eyes are red and watery. Then this morning we noticed a rash spreading all over his body.

病人家属：是我儿子，他已经病了几天了。他一直发高烧、咳嗽、流鼻涕、眼睛红且流泪。今天早上，我们发现他全身都长满了疹子。

**Doctor:** When did he start showing these symptoms?

医生：他什么时候开始出现这些症状的？

**Patient's family member:** He had a fever a few days ago, but the other symptoms started yesterday. The rash appeared this morning.

病人家属：他几天前开始发热，昨天开始出现其他症状，然后今天早上身上开始出现疹子。

**Doctor:** OK, I see. How old is your son?

医生：好的，了解。您的儿子多大了？

**Patient's family member:** He is two years old.

病人家属：两岁。

**Doctor:** Can you describe this rash to me?

医生：您可以描述一下他身上起的疹子吗？

**Patient's family member:** It started on his stomach then spread to his chest, back, arms and legs. The rash is red and bumpy.

病人家属：先起在肚子上，然后蔓延到胸口、背后、胳膊和腿上。疹子是红色凸起的。

> 🔍 **Key Words and Phrases**
>
> **bumpy** ['bʌmpi] adj. 不平的

**Doctor:** OK, we'll check on him.

医生：好的，我们给他检查一下。

*After examining.*

*检查后。*

**Doctor:** Can you tell me more about his medical history?

医生：您能告诉我更多关于他的病史吗？

**Patient's family member:** He's generally healthy and has got his vaccinations on time.

病人家属：他一直挺健康的，也都有按时接种疫苗。

**Doctor:** Has he been in contact with someone who has been diagnosed with measles recently?

医生：他最近有没有和被确诊为麻疹的人接触过？

**Patient's family member:** We're not very sure. Last weekend, we took him to an amusement park. Maybe some kids there have got measles.

病人家属：我们不太确定。上周末我们带他去了游乐园，也许那里有孩子感染了麻疹。

**Doctor:** Based on his symptoms and the appearance of the rash, I suspect he may have measles. We'll need to take him to the hospital for further evaluation and treatment.

医生：根据他的症状和皮疹的表现判断，我怀疑他可能得了麻疹。我们需要将他送往医院进行进一步评估和治疗。

**Patient's family member:** Measles? Is it serious?

病人家属：麻疹？那很严重吗？

**Doctor:** Measles is a highly contagious viral infection that can cause serious complications, especially in young children. That's why it's important to get him to the hospital as soon as possible.

医生：麻疹是一种传染性极强的病毒感染，尤其对年幼的孩子来说，麻疹能引起严重的并发症。所以我们需要尽快将他送到医院。

**Patient's family member:** OK, please help him.

病人家属：好的，请帮帮他。

**Doctor:** We'll do everything we can to help him. First, we need to take some protective measures to prevent the spread of the virus, such as wearing masks and isolating him from other people. Then, we'll give him a fever reducer to bring down the fever. We also need to provide him with oxygen so that he can breathe easier.

医生：我们会尽一切可能帮助他。首先，我们需要采取一些保护措施，防止病毒传播，例如戴口罩并采取隔离措施。然后，我们会给他服用退烧药来帮助退烧。我们还需要给他供氧，帮助他更顺畅地呼吸。

**Patient's family member:** Thank you so much. I'm really worried about him.

病人家属：非常感谢，我真的很担心他。

**Doctor:** I understand. We'll continue to monitor his vitals and make sure he gets the treatment he needs. Let's get him to the hospital now.

医生：我理解。我们会继续监测他的生命体征，确保他能得到所需的治疗。我们现在把他送去医院吧。

## Useful Expressions

What symptoms has the patient experienced?

病人有哪些症状？

When did the patient start showing these symptoms?

病人是什么时候开始出现这些症状的？

Is there a rash on the patient?

病人身上有起疹子吗？

Can you describe this rash to me?

您可以描述一下这种疹子吗？

Has the patient been in contact with someone who has been diagnosed with measles recently?

病人最近有没有和被确诊为麻疹的人接触过？

Has the patient injected a <u>measles vaccine</u>?

病人有没有注射过麻疹疫苗？

Based on the symptoms and the appearance of the rash, I suspect that the patient may have measles.

根据症状和皮疹的表现判断，我怀疑病人可能得了麻疹。

Measles is a highly contagious viral infection that can cause serious complications, especially in young children.

麻疹是一种传染性极强的病毒感染，尤其对年幼的孩子来说，麻疹能引起严重的并发症。

Measles typically begins with symptoms such as fever, cough, runny nose, and conjunctivitis before a rash develops.

麻疹通常先出现发热、咳嗽、流涕和结膜炎等症状，然后才会出现皮疹。

🔍 **Key Words and Phrases**

**measles vaccine** 麻疹疫苗

The rash usually starts on the face and spreads downward to the rest of the body.

皮疹通常从面部开始,向下蔓延到身体其他部位。

To prevent the spread of the virus, it's very important to isolate the patient from other people.

为了防止病毒传播,隔离病人是非常重要的。

The patient will need to be evaluated by a doctor and may require hospitalization.

病人需要接受医生的评估,还可能需要住院治疗。

## Section 2　Rabies
## 狂犬病

## Conversation

**Patient, male, 38 years old, was bitten on the leg by a stray dog one month ago. The patient cleaned the wound himself at home but did not seek medical attention promptly. Now the patient developed abnormal symptoms, and his family member immediately called for emergency medical services.**

病人,男性,38 岁,一个月前被一只流浪狗咬伤腿部。病人在家中自行清洗了伤口,但没有及时就医。现在病人出现了一些异常的症状,家属立即拨打了 120 急救电话。

**Doctor:** Hi, I'm a doctor from 120 Emergency. What seems to be the problem?

医生:您好! 我是 120 急救医生。请问发生了什么事?

**Patient's family member:** Hi, it is my brother. He has developed very strange symptoms these two days, like a fear of water and light, and difficulty swallowing.

病人家属：是我弟弟，他这两天出现了一些奇怪的症状，比如怕水、怕光，还有吞咽困难。

**Doctor:** Has he been bitten by an animal recently?

医生：他最近有被什么动物咬过吗？

**Patient's family member:** Yes, he was bitten by a stray dog a month ago.

病人家属：有，他一个月前被一只流浪狗咬伤了。

**Doctor:** Can you tell me more about the dog bite?

医生：关于那次被狗咬伤的经历，可以把详细情况再跟我说一下吗？

**Patient's family member:** Yes, the dog bit him on his leg. The wound was bleeding, and the surrounding skin was red, swollen and painful.

病人家属：好的。当时狗咬了他的腿部，伤口有流血，四周的皮肤红肿，还有疼痛。

**Doctor:** Was the wound cleaned thoroughly after the bite?

医生：他被咬后，有彻底清理伤口吗？

**Patient's family member:** My brother cleaned the wound himself at home, but he didn't seek medical attention promptly.

病人家属：他自己在家清洗了伤口，但是没有及时去医院。

**Doctor:** I see. If bitten by a dog, be sure to go to the hospital as soon as possible to prevent infection and other complications. Does he have other symptoms such as fever or headache?

医生：了解了。如果被狗咬了，一定要尽快去医院，防止发生感染和其他并发症。他还有没有其他症状？比如发热或头痛。

**Patient's family member:** Yes, he also has symptoms like fever and headache.

**病人家属：**有，他也出现了发热和头痛的症状。

**Doctor:** Is there any change in his behavior or mental state? For instance, unusually anxious or agitated?

医生：他的行为或精神状态是否有变化？比如表现出异常焦虑或不安。

**Patient's family member:** Yes, he seems to be very nervous.

**病人家属：**是的，他看起来很紧张。

*The doctor checks on the patient.*

*医生对病人进行检查。*

**Doctor:** Based on the symptoms, we suspect he may have rabies. Rabies is a serious disease that can be <u>transmitted</u> through <u>saliva</u>. It's important that we wear a mask and gloves, and put on protective clothing.

**医生：**根据症状判断，我们怀疑他感染了狂犬病。狂犬病是一种能够通过唾液传播的严重疾病。所以我们必须戴上口罩和手套，穿好防护服。

*The family members take necessary protective measures.*

*家属做好必要的防护措施。*

**Doctor:** We need to get him to the hospital right away for testing and treatment. The longer

> **🔍 Key Words and Phrases**
>
> **transmit** [trænzˈmɪt] v. 传播
> **saliva** [səˈlaɪvə] n. 唾液

the treatment is delayed, the lower chances of survival he will have. Does your brother have any medical conditions or allergies?

医生：我们必须立即送他到医院进行检查和治疗。治疗延误得越久，他生存的概率就越低。他有没有疾病史或过敏史？

**Patient's family member:** No.

病人家属：没有。

**Doctor:** Alright, we'll transport him to the hospital now. I'm going to give him a sedative to keep him calm on the way to the hospital. At the hospital, he will receive further medical care.

医生：好，那我们现在赶紧把他送到医院去。我会给他使用镇静剂，让他在去医院的路上保持平静。在医院，他将接受进一步的治疗。

**Patient's family member:** Thank you. Please save his life if possible.

病人家属：谢谢。请救救他。

**Doctor:** You're welcome. We'll take good care of him on the way to the hospital.

医生：不客气。在去医院的途中，我们会照顾好他。

## Useful Expressions

Has the patient been bitten by an animal recently?

病人最近被动物咬伤过吗？

Does the patient have any symptoms such as fever, headache, muscle weakness, or tingling around the area of the animal bite?

病人是否出现发热、头痛、肌肉无力或动物咬伤部位周围刺痛等症状？

Has the patient been experiencing any difficulty swallowing or an unusual fear of water or light?

病人有没有出现吞咽困难,异常畏水、畏光等症状?

Is there any change in the patient's behavior or mental state? For instance, unusually anxious or agitated?

病人的行为或精神状态是否有变化? 比如表现出异常焦虑或不安。

Has the patient been vaccinated against rabies?

病人是否接种过狂犬病疫苗?

Based on the symptoms and medical history, we suspect the patient may have rabies.

根据症状和病史判断,我们怀疑病人可能感染了狂犬病。

Rabies is a serious disease that can be transmitted through saliva. It's important that we wear a mask and gloves, and put on protective clothing.

狂犬病是一种能够通过唾液传播的严重疾病。所以我们必须戴上口罩和手套,穿好防护服。

I'm going to give the patient a sedative to keep him / her calm on the way to the hospital.

我会给病人使用镇静剂,让他 / 她在去医院的路上保持平静。

The patient will receive further medical care in hospital.

在医院,病人将会接受进一步的治疗。

# Section 3  Pulmonary Tuberculosis
# 肺结核

## Conversation

Patient, male, 35 years old, suddenly felt short of breath and began to cough violently, and coughed up a large amount of blood. His family member called for emergency medical services.

病人,男性,35 岁,突然感到呼吸困难,开始剧烈咳嗽,并咳出大量血液。家属拨打了 120 急救电话。

**Doctor:** Good evening, ma'am, I'm a paramedic. What's the situation here?

医生:晚上好,女士。我是急救医生,请问发生了什么事?

**Patient's family member:** It's my husband. He just started coughing violently and then there was a lot of blood.

病人家属:是我的丈夫,他刚刚突然急剧地咳嗽,然后咳了很多血。

**Doctor:** How much blood has he coughed up? Is it bright red or dark?

医生:他咳出了多少血,是鲜红色的还是暗红色的?

**Patient's family member:** It was a large amount of bright red

---

**🔍 Key Words and Phrases**

pulmonary tuberculosis 肺结核
short of breath 呼吸困难,气促

blood, like half a cup.

**病人家属**:他咳出了大量的鲜红色血液,差不多半杯那么多。

**Doctor:** Has he had any pain or tightness in his chest?

**医生**:他有没有胸痛或胸闷?

**Patient's family member:** Yes, he said he had chest pain and difficulty breathing.

**病人家属**:有,他说他胸口很痛,而且呼吸不过来。

**Doctor:** I see. Has he had any confirmed diseases?

**医生**:了解了,他有没有什么确诊的疾病?

**Patient's family member:** Not that we know of. He's usually quite fit and healthy. He doesn't even smoke.

**病人家属**:据我们所知应该是没有。他一直都挺健康的,也不吸烟。

**Doctor:** When did the coughing and shortness of breath start?

**医生**:他是什么时候开始咳嗽和呼吸困难的?

**Patient's family member:** For the past few months, he has been feeling tired and weak, and has also been experiencing symptoms such as coughing and fever.

**病人家属**:他最近几个月来一直感到疲劳、乏力,同时出现了咳嗽和发热的症状。

**Doctor:** Has he had any weight loss or loss of appetite recently?

**医生**:他近期有没有体重减轻或者食欲缺乏?

**Patient's family member:** Yes, he seemed to lose his appetite and weight these days.

**病人家属**:有,他看起来没什么胃口,体重也轻了。

**Doctor:** Has he experienced any night sweats?

医生：他有出现夜间盗汗吗？

**Patient's family member:** Yes, a lot. We assumed it was because of the hot weather.

病人家属：是的，出很多汗，我们都以为是天气太热的原因。

**Doctor:** Let me take a look at him. Sir, I'm going to check your breathing and oxygen levels. Try to take slow breaths for me.

医生：让我看看他的情况。先生，我要检查您的呼吸情况和血氧水平，请您尽量慢慢呼吸。

*The doctor examines the patient.*

*医生检查病人。*

**Doctor:** Based on the symptoms, I suspect that your husband may have pulmonary tuberculosis.

医生：根据症状判断，我怀疑您的丈夫可能患上了肺结核。

**Patient's family member:** Is it serious?

病人家属：这种病严重吗？

**Doctor:** Pulmonary tuberculosis is a chronic infectious disease. He will be OK if treated promptly. First, we need to take protective measures to prevent the possible spread of tuberculosis to others.

医生：肺结核是一种慢性传染病，如果治疗及时，您丈夫应该会没事的。首先，我们需要采取保护措施，防止结核病传播。

**Patient's family member:** What should we do?

病人家属：我们应该怎么做？

**Doctor:** We all need to wear masks and gloves, and the patient will be isolated from others during the transport. Also, you and anyone who has been in close contact with him should also get tested for tuberculosis.

医生：我们所有人都需要戴上口罩和手套。在转运过程中，我们还要隔离病人。还有，您和与他有过密切接触的人员都需要接受结核检查。

**Patient's family member:** OK, thank you for letting us know.

病人家属：好的，谢谢您告诉我们。

**Doctor:** We're going to start oxygen and an intravenous injection. Let's get him transported as soon as possible. If the patient has massive hemoptysis during transportation, we may intubate the trachea if necessary.

医生：我们要为他提供氧气和静脉注射，并尽快把他送到医院去。如果在转运期间病人出现大量咯血，必要时我们可能要对他进行气管插管。

**Patient's family member:** Thank you. We'll meet you at the hospital.

病人家属：谢谢。我们会在医院跟你们会合。

**Doctor:** No problem, we'll do everything we can for him.

医生：不客气，我们会尽全力帮助他的。

## Useful Expressions

When did the coughing and shortness of breath start?

咳嗽和呼吸困难是什么时候开始的？

Has the patient been coughing up blood?

病人有咳血吗？

How much blood has the patient coughed up? Is it bright red or dark?

病人咳出了多少血,是鲜红色的还是暗红色的?

Has the patient had any pain or tightness in the chest?

病人有没有胸痛或者胸闷?

Has the patient had any weight loss or loss of appetite recently?

病人近期有没有体重减轻或者食欲缺乏?

Has the patient experienced any night sweat?

病人有没有夜间盗汗的情况?

Let me listen to your lungs. Take deep breaths.

让我听听您的肺部,深呼吸。

Does the patient have a history of pulmonary tuberculosis?

病人有没有肺结核病史?

Based on the symptoms, we suspect that the patient may have pulmonary tuberculosis.

根据症状判断,我们怀疑病人可能患有肺结核。

We'll need to take protective measures to prevent the possible spread of tuberculosis to others.

我们需要采取保护措施,防止结核病传播。

## Section 4　Tetanus
### 破伤风

## Conversation

Patient, female, 25 years old, had symptoms of clenched jaw, difficult swallowing and

**Key Words and Phrases**

clench [klentʃ] v. 咬紧
jaw [dʒɔː] n. 下巴;v. 闲谈,唠唠叨叨

**breathing at home. Her family called for emergency medical services.**

病人，女性，25 岁，在家中出现牙关紧闭、吞咽困难、呼吸困难等症状，家属拨打了 120 急救电话。

**Doctor:** Hello, I'm Dr. Han. Can you tell me what happened?

医生：您好，我是韩医生。请问发生了什么事？

**Patient's family member:** It is my daughter. This morning she suddenly felt unwell. She couldn't open her mouth, had trouble swallowing and sometimes couldn't breathe. I got so scared seeing her like this that I called 120 immediately.

病人家属：是我女儿，她今天早上突然感觉不舒服。她张不开嘴巴，吞咽有困难，有时候甚至无法呼吸。看到她这样我吓坏了，所以立刻拨打了 120 急救电话。

**Doctor:** Has she had any recent wounds, cuts or <u>punctures</u>?

医生：她最近有没有受过伤？比如割伤或刺伤。

**Patient's family member:** Yes, she cut her finger 5 days ago and just had a fever 2 days ago.

病人家属：有的，她 5 天前割伤了手指，2 天前还发热了。

**Doctor:** Does she have any other symptoms, such as sweating, high blood pressure, or <u>accelerated</u> heartbeat?

医生：她有没有出现其他症状？比如出汗、高血压或心跳加速。

**Patient's family member:** Yes, she has been sweating continuously and her heartbeat

---

**🔍 Key Words and Phrases**

**puncture** ['pʌŋktʃə] n. 刺伤

**accelerated** [æk'seləreɪtɪd] adj. 加速的

is a little fast.

病人家属：有，她一直都在出汗，心跳也有点快。

**Doctor:** I see. Based on her symptoms, it seems she may have tetanus. Let me examine her quickly. Has she had tetanus vaccination before?

医生：我了解了。根据她的症状判断，可能是破伤风。让我快速检查一下，她之前接种过破伤风疫苗吗？

**Patient's family member:** Tetanus? I don't think she ever had that vaccination.

病人家属：破伤风？她应该没有接种过。

**Doctor:** Can you tell me if she has any other medical conditions or takes any medications regularly?

医生：请问她是否有其他疾病，常吃什么药？

**Patient's family member:** No, she's very healthy.

病人家属：没有，她挺健康的。

**Doctor:** Alright, that's helpful to know. I'm giving her some medications to relieve the muscle spasms first. And my colleague will wrap a tongue depressor with gauze and place it between her upper and lower molars to prevent tongue biting. And then we will get her on a stretcher and take her to the hospital. We need to let her lie on her side to prevent aspiration in case of vomiting.

医生：好的，知道这些对我们很有帮助。我先给她使用一些药物来舒缓肌肉痉挛，我的同事会在她的上下磨牙之间放一个裹了纱布的压舌板，防止她咬伤舌头。然后我们会把她抬上担架，送去医院，我们要让她保持侧卧位，防止误吸呕吐物。

**Patient's family member:** OK, thank you so much.

**病人家属:**好的,谢谢你们。

*The doctor and nurse transport the patient into the ambulance.*

急救人员将病人转运到救护车上。

**Doctor:** Now we're going to provide oxygen and intravenous injection fluids for her. We'll be monitoring her condition closely during the transport.

**医生:**现在我们准备为她供氧和进行静脉输液。我们会在转运过程中密切监测她的病情。

**Patient's family member:** Thank you. Please take good care of my daughter!

**病人家属:**谢谢。请一定照顾好我女儿!

**Doctor:** We absolutely will.

**医生:**我们一定会的。

## Useful Expressions

Has the patient had any recent wounds, cuts or punctures?

病人最近有没有受过伤? 比如割伤或刺伤。

Is the patient experiencing <u>muscle stiffness</u>, spasms, or difficulty breathing?

病人是否出现肌肉僵硬、痉挛或呼吸困难?

When did the patient's jaw first start feeling tight or have difficulty opening?

病人是什么时候开始感到牙关紧绷或打不开的?

Does the patient have any other symptoms, such as sweating, high blood pressure,

> **Key Words and Phrases**
>
> **muscle stiffness** <医> 肌强直

or accelerated heartbeat?

病人有没有出现其他症状? 比如出汗、高血压或心跳加速。

Based on the symptoms, we suspect that the patient may have tetanus.

根据症状判断,我们怀疑病人可能感染了破伤风。

Has the patient had tetanus vaccination before?

病人有没有接种过破伤风疫苗?

If the patient has any other medical conditions or takes any medications regularly?

病人是否有其他疾病,常吃什么药?

We'll give the patient a sedative to help relax his / her muscles and prevent spasms during transport.

我们会给病人使用镇静剂以帮助放松肌肉,并在转运过程中防止痉挛。

We'll provide the patient with oxygen to help with his / her breathing and start an intravenous infusion.

我们将为病人提供氧气来帮助呼吸,并开始静脉输液。

# Unit 7

## Common Traumas
## 常见创伤

### Section 1　Traffic Accident Injury
### 交通伤

#### Conversation

Patient, female, 28 years old, had injuries in a traffic accident. Some witnesses called for emergency medical services.

病人，女性，28 岁，在一起车祸中受伤，目击者拨打了 120 急救电话。

**Doctor:** Ma'am, I'm an EMT. Can you hear me?

医生：女士，我是急救医生，您能听见我说话吗？

**Patient:** Yes.

病人：能。

**Doctor:** Now I am going to assess your injuries, please try to keep still.

医生：我现在要评估一下您的伤势，请尽量不要动。

*The doctor checks the patient's vital signs by using the ABCDE assessment.*

医生对病人进行了 ABCDE 生命体征评估。

**Doctor:** Ma'am, your breathing is rapid and shallow, your pulse is very fast, and your blood pressure is quite low. I will provide oxygen to help you breathe and start an intravenous injection. And you are bleeding, so my colleague is going to stop the bleeding for you.

医生:女士,您的呼吸急促且微弱,脉搏很快,血压很低。我现在为您供氧,帮助您呼吸,同时为您进行静脉注射。您还在流血,我同事会帮您止血。

*The doctor and nurse perform necessary medical cares for the patient.*

急救人员对病人进行急救护理。

**Doctor:** I will gently press the area to check if there is swelling, bruising or tenderness. Let me know if you feel any pain anywhere.

医生:我会轻轻按压伤处,检查有无肿胀、挫伤或触痛。如果有地方感到疼痛请告知我。

**Patient:** OK.

病人:好的。

**Doctor:** Now I'm going to check your arms and legs for any deformity or discoloration which could indicate a fracture.

医生:我现在要检查您的

**🔍 Key Words and Phrases**

**bruising** [ˈbruːzɪŋ] n. 挫伤

**tenderness** [ˈtendənɪs] n. 触痛

**deformity** [dɪˈfɔːməti] n. 畸形

**discoloration** [dɪsˌkʌləˈreɪʃən] n. 变色

**fracture** [ˈfræktʃə(r)] n. 骨折

手脚，看看有无畸形或发暗的情况，这可能预示着骨折。

**Patient:** My left leg really hurts.

病人：我左腿非常痛。

**Doctor:** You may have a fracture on your left leg. I will put a <u>splint</u> on it to prevent further damage.

医生：您的左腿可能骨折了。我用夹板帮您固定住，防止进一步损伤。

**Patient:** OK, thank you.

病人：好的，谢谢。

**Doctor:** To check if you have suffered a <u>concussion</u> in the accident, I'm going to ask you some questions to check your memory and <u>cognitive function</u>. Can you tell me your name and age?

医生：为了检查您在事故中是否发生了脑震荡，我要问您一些问题，检查您的记忆和认知功能。您能告诉我您的名字和年龄吗？

**Patient:** My name is Jane. And I'm 28.

病人：我叫简，28 岁。

**Doctor:** Can you tell me the details of the accident?

医生：您能跟我说说事故的详细经过吗？

**Patient:** Yes. I was riding a bike and going through an

---

🔍 **Key Words and Phrases**

**splint** [splɪnt] n.（固定骨折的）夹板

**concussion** [kənˈkʌʃn] n. 脑震荡，震荡，冲击，震动

**cognitive function** 认知功能

intersection. A car came out from my left side and bumped into me directly. I fell off my bike.

病人:好的。我当时骑着自行车,穿过一个十字路口的时候,一辆小汽车突然从我的左边驶出,直接撞上了我,我从自行车上摔了下来。

**Doctor:** Did you hit your head when you fell?

医生:您落地的时候是否撞到了头?

**Patient:** Yes. My head hit the pavement a little bit.

病人:有,我的头在人行道上撞了一下。

**Doctor:** I need to immobilize your neck and spine as a precaution until we can rule out any fractures or spinal injuries.

医生:在排除骨折和脊柱损伤之前,我需要固定您的脖子和脊柱,以防万一。

**Patient:** OK

病人:好的。

**Doctor:** We need to get you to the hospital as soon as possible to get a full examination including imaging examination. Just try to remain as still as you can.

医生:我们需要尽快把您送到医院进行全面检查,包括影像学检查。请尽量保持不动。

**Patient:** OK, thank you.

病人:好的,谢谢。

## Useful Expressions

Can you hear me?

> 🔍 **Key Words and Phrases**
>
> **intersection** [ˌɪntəˈsekʃn] n. 十字路口
> **bump into** 撞上,偶然碰见
> **fall off** 跌落
> **pavement** [ˈpeɪvmənt] n. 人行道
> **spine** [spaɪn] n. 脊柱
> **spinal** [ˈspaɪnl] adj. 脊柱的

您能听到我说话吗？

I will gently press the area to check if there is swelling, bruising or tenderness. Let me know if anything hurts.

我会轻轻按压伤处，检查有无肿胀、挫伤或触痛。如果感到疼痛请告知我。

I'm going to check your arms and legs for any deformity or discoloration which could indicate a fracture.

我要检查您的手脚，看看有无畸形或发暗的情况，这可能预示着骨折。

I will put a splint on your… (body part) to prevent further damage.

我将用夹板固定您的……（身体部位），防止进一步受伤。

To check if you have suffered a concussion in the accident, I'm going to ask you some questions to check your memory and cognitive function.

为了检查您在事故中是否发生了脑震荡，我要问您一些问题，检查您的记忆和认知功能。

Can you tell me your name and age?

您能告诉我您的名字和年龄吗？

Can you tell me the details of the accident?

您能跟我说说事故的详细经过吗？

I need to immobilize your neck / spine as a precaution until we can rule out any fractures or spinal injuries.

在排除骨折和脊柱损伤之前，我需要固定您的脖子／脊柱，以防万一。

We need to get you to the hospital as soon as possible to get a full examination, including imaging examination.

我们需要尽快把您送到医院进行全面检查,包括影像学检查。

Just try to remain as still as you can.

请尽量保持不动。

# Section 2  Injury by Falling from Height
# 坠落伤

## Conversation

**Patient, male, 35 years old, fell from a <u>scaffolding</u>. His family member called for emergency medical services.**

病人,男性,35 岁,从脚手架上跌落,家属拨打了 120 急救电话。

**Doctor:** Hi there, my name is Li Hua and I'm a paramedic. Can you tell me your name?

医生:您好! 我叫李华,是一名急救医生。您能告诉我您的名字吗?

**Patient:** My name is Jack.

病人:我叫杰克。

**Doctor:** OK, Jack, try to stay calm. Can you tell me how did you fall?

医生:好的,杰克。请尽量保持冷静。您能告诉我您是怎么摔下来的吗?

---

🔍 **Key Words and Phrases**

**scaffolding** [ˈskæfəldɪŋ] n.
脚手架

---

**Patient:** I was working on a scaffolding about 3 meters up. The scaffolding came loose and I lost my balance and fell off, landing on the <u>cement</u> ground below.

病人：我站在一个大概 3m 高的脚手架上干活，脚手架突然松了，我失去了平衡，摔了下来，直接摔到了水泥地板上。

**Doctor:** Alright, I'm going to do a quick assessment to check for any injuries. Do you feel any pain in your neck, chest, back, or limbs?

医生：好的。我要快速评估一下您的伤情。您的颈部、胸部、背部或四肢是否感到疼痛？

**Patient:** Yes, my ribs hurt when I breathe. It's really hard to take a deep breath.

病人：有，呼吸的时候，我的肋骨会很痛，很难深呼吸。

**Doctor:** It sounds like you may have some broken ribs. I'm going to listen to your breathing. Just try to relax.

医生：好的，看起来您可能是肋骨骨折了。我要听一下您的呼吸。尽量放松。

*The doctor checks the patient's breathing.*

*医生检查病人的呼吸。*

**Patient:** My back is killing me too. I landed straight on my back. It really hurts to move.

病人：我的背部也很痛。落地的时候是背部直接着地的，太痛了，根本动不了。

**Doctor:** Did you lose consciousness at any point during the fall?

医生：坠落期间您有失去意识吗？

> 🔍 **Key Words and Phrases**
>
> **cement** [sɪˈment] n. 水泥；v. 巩固，加强，使黏结

**Patient:** No, but I feel very

dizzy right now.

病人:没有,但是我现在觉得头晕。

**Doctor:** You might have a head trauma or concussion if you experience symptoms like dizziness, headache, or confusion. We need to transport you to hospital for further evaluation and treatment. I'm going to gently press on different areas of your body to check for internal bleeding or organ damage. Let me know if you feel any pain.

医生:如果出现头晕、头痛或意识混乱等症状,很可能有头部创伤或发生了脑震荡。我们需要将您送往医院进行进一步评估和治疗。我将轻轻按压您身体的不同部位,以检查是否有内出血或器官损伤。如果您感到疼痛,请告诉我。

**Patient:** OK, thank you.

病人:好的,谢谢。

**Doctor:** As precaution, we may need to immobilize your neck and spine. I know it's uncomfortable, but try to remain still while we secure you to the stretcher and get you into the ambulance. I'm going to give you some pain relief to help you feel better.

医生:为谨慎起见,我们可能需要固定您的颈部和脊柱。我知道会很不舒服,但在我们将您固定到担架上,送进救护车之前,请尽量保持不动。我会给您开一些止痛药,让您感觉舒服些。

**Nurse:** Alright, I'm going to start an intravenous injection to give you some pain medications and fluids.

护士:好的,我现在为您进行静脉注射,注入一些止痛药并进行补液。

**Patient:** OK, thank you for your help.

病人：好的，谢谢你们的帮助。

**Doctor:** Can you tell me if you have any allergies or medical conditions?

医生：请问您有没有过敏史或疾病史？

**Patient:** No, I don't have any allergies or medical conditions.

病人：没有，我没有过敏史或疾病史。

**Doctor:** OK, good to know. We'll be at the hospital soon, and the doctors will assess your injuries further and get you treated.

医生：好的，了解。我们很快就会到医院，那里的医生会为您进行进一步评估和治疗。

**Patient:** Thank you, I appreciate it.

病人：谢谢，我很感激。

## Useful Expressions

Can you tell me how did you fall?

请问您是怎么摔下来的？

I'm going to do a quick assessment to check for any injuries.

我要快速评估一下您的伤情。

Do you feel any pain in your neck, chest, back, or limbs?

您的颈部、胸部、背部或四肢是否感到疼痛？

I'm going to listen to your breathing. Just try to relax.

我要听一下您的呼吸。尽量放松。

Did you lose consciousness at any point during the fall?

坠落期间您有失去意识吗？

You might have a head trauma or concussion if you experience symptoms like dizziness, headache, or confusion.

如果出现头晕、头痛或意识混乱等症状，很可能有头部创伤或发生了脑震荡。

As precaution, we may need to immobilize your neck and spine.

为谨慎起见，我们可能需要固定您的颈部和脊柱。

I know it's uncomfortable, but try to remain still while we secure you to the stretcher and get you into the ambulance.

我知道会很不舒服，但在我们将您固定到担架上，送进救护车之前，请尽量保持不动。

I'm going to give you some pain relief to help you feel better.

我会给您开一些止痛药，让您感觉舒服些。

Can you tell me if you have any allergies or medical conditions?

您有没有过敏史或疾病史？

## Section 3　Mechanical Injury
## 机械伤

### Conversation

Patient, male, 45 years old, accidentally got his right hand caught in the machinery while operating a machine at a factory, and his wrist was stuck and unable to be pulled out.

🔍 **Key Words and Phrases**

mechanical [məˈkænɪkl] adj. 机械（学）的
machinery [məˈʃiːnəri] n. 机器
wrist [rɪst] n. 手腕，腕关节
pull out 拔出，退出

**His colleague called for emergency medical services**

病人,男性,45 岁,在工厂操作机器时,右手不小心卷入机器,手腕部分被卡住,无法取出。他的同事拨打了 120 急救电话。

**Doctor:** Hi there, my name is Li Hua and I'm a doctor. Can you tell me your name and how did you get your hand caught in the machine?

医生:您好! 我叫李华,是一名医生。您能告诉我您的名字以及您的手是怎么被机器卡住的吗?

**Patient:** My name is Mike. I was operating a machine, then my right hand got caught between two <u>gears</u>. I couldn't pull it out, and my wrist is stuck.

病人:我叫迈克。我刚才在操作一台机器,突然我的右手被卷进了两个齿轮中,没办法拔出来,我的手腕被卡住了。

**Doctor:** Alright, try not to panic. I'm checking your hand for broken bones, <u>dislocations</u>, and soft <u>tissue</u> damage. Please let me know if anything hurts.

医生:好的,请尽量不要惊慌。我要检查一下您的手是否有骨折、脱位和软组织损伤。如果觉得痛,请您告诉我。

*The doctor examines the patient's hand.*

医生检查病人的手。

**Doctor:** It looks like you have <u>lacerations</u> and soft tissue damage. There may also be fractures or nerve injuries. Can

> **🔍 Key Words and Phrases**
>
> **gear** [gɪə] n. 齿轮
> **dislocation** [dɪsləˈkeɪʃn] n. 脱臼
> **tissue** [ˈtɪʃuː] n.(动植物的)组织
> **laceration** [læsəˈreɪʃn] n. 撕裂

you tell me how much pain you're feeling right now?

医生:看起来有割伤和软组织损伤,还可能有骨折或神经受损。您能告诉我您现在的疼痛程度吗?

**Patient:** The pain is intermittent, but when it comes, it's intense.

病人:疼痛断断续续的,但当疼痛来临时,非常剧烈。

**Doctor:** There is a closed soft tissue <u>contusion</u> and part of your palm's soft tissue is torn. There's also a lot of bleeding. Once we release your wrist from the gears, we need to stop the bleeding and stabilize the injured area to prevent further damage.

医生:您的手腕有闭合性软组织挫伤,手掌部分软组织被撕裂,出了很多血。一旦将您的手腕从齿轮中移出,我们需要立刻止血并固定受伤部位,防止进一步损伤。

*The emergency staff successfully releases the patient's wrist from the gears.*

*急救人员成功将病人的手腕从齿轮中移出。*

**Doctor:** Alright. I'm going to apply a <u>tourniquet</u> to stop the bleeding. It will hurt a little.

医生:我要使用<u>止血带</u>帮您止血。这可能会有点儿疼。

**Patient:** It's OK.

病人:没关系。

**Doctor:** Now we need to get you to the hospital for further treatment. I'm going to give you some pain medications through intravenous injection. It will help reduce your pain and

> **🔍 Key Words and Phrases**
>
> **contusion** [kən'tjuːʒn] n. 挫伤
>
> **tourniquet** ['tʊənɪkeɪ] n. 止血带

discomfort. Can you tell me if you have any allergies or medical conditions?

医生：我们需要将您送往医院接受进一步治疗。我将为您静脉注射止痛药，这有助于减轻您的疼痛和不适。您能告诉我您是否有过敏史或疾病史吗？

**Patient:** No.

病人：没有。

**Doctor:** Great. We're going to transport you to the hospital now. It's very important that you stay still. Any unnecessary movement could worsen your condition.

医生：好的。我们现在将把您送往医院。请务必保持不动。任何不必要的移动都可能使您的状况恶化。

**Patient:** OK, thank you for your help.

病人：好的，谢谢你们的帮助。

## Useful Expressions

Can you tell me your name and how did you get your... (body part) caught in the machine?

您能告诉我您的名字以及您的……（身体部位）是怎么被机器卡住的吗？

I'm checking for broken bones, dislocations, and soft tissue damage. Please let me know if anything hurts.

我要检查一下是否有骨折、脱位和软组织损伤。如果觉得痛，请您告诉我。

It looks like you have lacerations and soft tissue damage. There may also be fractures or nerve injuries.

看起来您有割伤和软组织损伤,还可能有骨折或神经受损。

Can you tell me how much pain you're feeling right now?

您能告诉我您现在的疼痛程度吗?

I need to stabilize the injured area to prevent further damage.

我需要固定受伤部位,防止进一步损伤。

I'm going to apply a tourniquet to stop the bleeding. It will hurt a little.

我要使用止血带帮您止血。这可能会有点儿疼。

I'm going to give you some pain medications through intravenous injection. It will help reduce your pain and discomfort.

我将为您静脉注射止痛药,这有助于减轻您的疼痛和不适。

It's very important that you stay still. Any unnecessary movement could worsen your condition.

请务必保持不动。任何不必要的移动都可能使您的状况恶化。

## Section 4　Sharp Instrument Injury
### 锐器伤

### Conversation

Patient, male, 25 years old, was stabbed by a drunken stranger with a knife on the street. A witness called for

**Q Key Words and Phrases**

sharp [ʃɑːp] adj. 锋利的

instrument [ˈɪnstrəmənt] n. 器械

stab [stæb] v. 刺

drunken [ˈdrʌŋkən] adj. 醉的

**emergency medical services.**

病人，男性，25 岁，在街上被陌生醉汉持刀刺伤。一位目击者拨打了 120 急救电话。

**Doctor:** Hi there, my name is Li Hua and I'm a doctor. Can you tell me your name?

医生：您好，我是李华，是一名医生。您能告诉我您的名字吗?

**Patient:** My name is Alex.

病人：我叫亚历克斯。

**Doctor:** OK, Alex. I'm going to check your wound now.

医生：亚历克斯，我现在要检查一下您的伤口。

*The doctor examines the wounds.*

*医生检查伤口。*

**Doctor:** It looks like you have multiple stab wounds on your left side. I'm going to apply pressure to check how deep the wound is. This may hurt a bit. Take slow, deep breaths for me.

医生：看起来您左侧身体有多处刺伤，我现在要按压看看伤口有多深，这可能会有点儿痛。请慢慢深呼吸。

**Patient:** Ah! It hurts when you press there.

病人：啊，您按压的时候很痛。

**Doctor:** I know, I'm sorry. But we need to slow the bleeding. I'm going to wrap some bandages around your chest and arm now to help control bleeding. Alex, do you still remember what happened?

> **🔍 Key Words and Phrases**
>
> **multiple** [ˈmʌltɪpl] adj. 多重的

**医生:**我知道会很痛,非常抱歉,但是我们需要减缓出血。我现在要对您的胸部和手臂进行包扎,以控制出血。亚历克斯,您还记得发生了什么吗?

**Patient:** I was taking a walk on the street, and suddenly a drunk guy came out from nowhere and he stabbed me with a knife. I was stabbed on my left side, on my ribs, upper arm and hand.

**病人:**我在街上散步的时候,有个喝醉的家伙不知道从哪里冒出来,拿刀刺伤了我。我左侧的肋骨、上臂和手都被刺伤了。

**Doctor:** I am sorry to hear that. Are you feeling lightheaded or dizzy?

**医生:**很抱歉听到您遇到了这样的事。您是否感到头晕或眩晕?

**Patient:** Yes, a little. Maybe it's because of the bleeding.

**病人:**有点儿,可能是因为流血了吧。

**Doctor:** We need to get you to the hospital as soon as possible. Can you tell me if you have any allergies or medical conditions?

**医生:**我们现在要尽快将您送到医院去。您有过敏史或疾病史吗?

**Patient:** No, I don't have any allergies or medical conditions.

**病人:**没有,我没有过敏史或疾病史。

**Doctor:** OK, great. We're going to transport you to the nearest hospital now. We'll provide oxygen and start an intravenous injection to give you some pain relief. And we'll continue to monitor your vital signs on the way there.

**医生:**好的。我们现在要把您转送到最近的医院。我们会为您供氧,静脉注射一些止痛药。在去医院的路上,我们会继续监测您的生命体征。

**Patient:** Thank you for your help.

**病人:** 谢谢你们的帮助。

**Doctor:** You're welcome.

**医生:** 不客气。

## Useful Expressions

Were you stabbed by a sharp object?

您是被什么锐器刺到了吗?

It looks like you have multiple stab wounds.

看起来您有多处刺伤。

I'm going to check your wound now.

我现在要检查一下您的伤口。

I'm going to apply pressure to check how deep the wound is.
This may hurt a bit.

我现在要按压看看伤口有多深,这可能会有点儿痛。

I'm going to wrap some bandages around your… (body part)
now to help control bleeding.

我现在要对您的……(身体部位)进行包扎,以控制出血。

Are you feeling lightheaded or dizzy?

您是否感到头晕或眩晕?

Do you have chills, fever, or other signs of infection?

您是否出现了寒战、发热或其他感染的迹象?

Has the area around the wound become red or swollen?

伤口周围的区域是否变红或肿胀?

I'm going to clean the wound and dress it to prevent infection.

我现在要清洁并包扎伤口,预防感染。

We need to get you to the hospital for specialized treatment, including stitching.

我们需要把您送去医院,进行包括缝合在内的专业治疗。

# Section 5　Injury from a Low Fall or Collision
# 跌撞伤

## Conversation

**Patient, female, 70 years old, fell down accidentally while walking at home, feeling severe pain in the head and chest and unable to stand up on her own. Her family member immediately called for emergency medical services.**

病人,女性,70 岁,在家中走路时不慎摔倒,感到头部和胸口非常疼痛,无法自行站起,家属立即拨打了 120 急救电话。

**Doctor:** Hello, I'm a doctor from 120 Emergency. Can you tell me what happened? How did the patient fall?

医生:您好,我是 120 急救医生。您能告诉我发生了什么事吗,病人是怎么摔倒的?

**Patient's family member:** My grandmother is 70 years old. This morning, when she was walking around the house, she slipped and fell.

病人家属:我奶奶已经 70 岁了。她今天在家里走路的

> **Key Words and Phrases**
>
> collision [kəˈlɪʒn] n. 碰撞,冲突
> stand up on one's own 自己站起来
> slip [slɪp] v. 滑

时候不小心滑倒了。

**Doctor:** What were her symptoms after the fall?

医生：她摔倒之后有什么症状？

**Patient's family member:** She said she hit her head and chest on the floor and now she's in a lot of pain. We tried to help her stand up but she couldn't get up on her own.

病人家属：她说她的头和胸部撞到地板了，现在非常痛。我们想帮她站起来，可是她没办法自行站立起来。

**Doctor:** OK, don't try to move her. Did she lose consciousness after the fall?

医生：好的，请不要移动她。病人摔倒后有没有失去知觉？

**Patient's family member:** No, she's been awake but she seems very disoriented and confused.

病人家属：没有，她还清醒着，但她看起来好像非常迷茫和困惑。

**Doctor:** Alright, we'll need to get her to the hospital right away. I'm going to examine her vitals now. Can you tell me if she's complained of any other pains or symptoms?

医生：好的。我们现在要立刻把她送到医院去。我现在要给她测量一下生命体征。您能告诉我她有没有提及其他的疼痛或症状吗？

**Patient's family member:** She said her chest really hurts when she tries to take a deep breath. And she feels dizzy any time we tried to lift her up. Oh, and she said her head is killing her.

病人家属：她说她深呼吸的

> 🔍 **Key Words and Phrases**
>
> **lift sb. up** 扶起某人

时候胸口会痛。我们试着把她扶起来时,她说觉得头晕。哦,她还说她的头剧痛无比。

**Doctor:** OK, these are all possible symptoms from a fall like this. Can you tell me if she has any allergies or medical conditions?

医生:好的,这些都是跌倒后可能会出现的症状。您能告诉我她是否有过敏史或疾病史吗?

**Patient's family member:** She has some other health issues like high blood pressure, and she is allergic to penicillin.

病人家属:她有高血压,而且对青霉素过敏。

**Doctor:** OK, get it. We're going to get her to the hospital as soon as we can to check for any fractures or internal bleeding. We're going to put a neck brace on her and a spine board behind her to prevent further harm. We'll also put a blood pressure cuff on her arm and a pulse <u>oximeter</u> on her finger to monitor her vital signs. One of you can ride with us to the hospital.

医生:好的,了解。我们现在要尽快把她送到医院,检查有没有骨折或内出血。我们会给她戴上颈托,并在她身后放置一个脊柱固定板,防止进一步的伤害。我们还会在她的手臂上放置血压袖带,在她的手指上夹上脉搏血氧仪,监测她的生命体征。你们有一位家属可以跟车去医院。

**Patient's family member:** Yes of course, thank you so much.

病人家属:好的,非常感谢。

**Doctor:** We'll do everything we can.

医生:我们一定会尽力的。

> **🔍 Key Words and Phrases**
>
> **oximeter** [ɒkˈsɪmɪtə] n. 血氧(定量)计

## Useful Expressions

*For the family member:*

*向家属提问：*

How did the patient fall?

病人是怎么摔倒的？

What were the patient's symptoms after the fall?

病人摔倒之后有什么症状？

Where does the patient feel the pain?

病人哪个部位疼痛？

Did the patient lose consciousness after the fall?

病人摔倒后有没有失去知觉？

*For the patient:*

*向病人提问：*

Do you feel any numbness or tingling in your arms or legs?

您的手或脚是否有麻木或刺痛感？

Do you feel any pain when you move your... (body part) ?

您在动您的……（身体部位）的时候会觉得痛吗？

Did you hit your head during the fall or collision?

您在摔倒或碰伤的时候有没有撞到头部？

Do you have any cuts or bruises?

您有没有割伤或擦伤？

Let me check your... (body part) for any swelling or deformity.

让我检查一下您的……（身体部位）有没有肿胀或畸形。

I'm going to gently press on different areas, please let me

know if it hurts.

我要轻轻按压不同的部位,如果有部位感到疼痛,请告知我。

Are you having difficulty breathing?

您呼吸困难吗?

Can you stand up and walk without assistance?

您能自主站立行走吗?

Are you feeling dizzy or lightheaded?

您有没有眩晕或头晕?

Have you taken any medications or consumed alcohol recently?

您最近有没有服用药物或饮酒?

I'm going to stabilize your... (body part) to minimize movement for now, just as a precaution.

为谨慎起见,我现在要固定您的……(身体部位)以减少行动。

## Section 6　Firearm Injury
## 火器伤

### Conversation

**Patient, male, 34 years old, was shot in the chest and was in a coma. A witness called for emergency medical services.**

病人,男性,34岁,被枪击中胸部,处于昏迷状态。一名目击

🔍 **Key Words and Phrases**

firearm ['faɪərɑːm] n. 火器

shoot [ʃuːt] v. 射击;n. 射击,镜头,注射

者拨打了 120 急救电话。

Upon arriving at the scene, the emergency doctor checked the man's vital signs and found that he had stopped breathing and had no heartbeat. The emergency personnel immediately began cardiopulmonary resuscitation, providing chest compressions and artificial respiration, while also activating the automated external defibrillator (AED) for defibrillation. After three rounds of defibrillation, the man's heartbeat was restored, but he still did not regain consciousness. The emergency personnel quickly lifted the man onto a stretcher and performed tracheal intubation and assisted breathing with a ventilator, while also providing supportive treatments such as intravenous fluids and pain relief.

到达事故现场后,急救医生检查了该男子的生命体征,发现其已经停止呼吸、心跳。急救人员立刻进行了心肺复苏,给予胸外心脏按压和人工呼吸,同时开启自动体外除颤仪进行除颤。经过 3 次除颤后,男子的心跳恢复,但仍未恢复自主意识。急救人员迅速将男子抬上担架,进行气管插管和呼吸机辅助呼吸,同时给予静脉输液、止痛等支持治疗。

**Doctor:** Sir, can you tell me exactly what happened here?

医生:先生,您能告诉我到底发生了什么事吗?

**Witness:** We were all just standing around talking after work when this guy in a hoodie and mask came up and started shooting. He shot that man multiple times in the chest and then ran off that way.

**目击者:**我们当时刚下班,站在路边聊天,突然有个穿着连帽衫、戴着口罩的人跑出来,并开始射击。他朝那个人的胸部开了好几枪,然后就立刻跑掉了。

**Doctor:** OK, do you know the victim's name or any medical history?

**医生:**好的,您知道伤者的名字或者医疗史吗?

**Witness:** His name is John, I think he works at the company across the street. I don't know anything about his medical history.

**目击者:**他叫约翰,应该在街道对面那家公司工作,我不了解他的医疗史。

**Doctor:** Did you notice any other injuries on the victim besides the gunshot wound to his chest?

**医生:**除了他胸部的枪伤,您有没有注意到伤者身上是否有其他伤?

**Witness:** No, I didn't see any other injuries. He was bleeding pretty heavily from the chest, though.

**目击者:**没有,我没有看到其他的伤口,但是他的胸部流了很多血。

**Doctor:** Thank you for your help. We'll be sure to include your statement in our report. Is there anything else you can tell us that might be helpful?

**医生:**谢谢您的帮忙。我们会把您提供的信息记录在报告里。还有其他您觉得有用的信息吗?

**Witness:** No, that's all I saw. I just hope the man is going to be OK.

**目击者:**没有了,我看到的只有这些了。我只希望那个人没事。

**Doctor:** We'll do everything we can to help him. Thanks again for your assistance.

医生:我们会尽力救治他。再次感谢您的协助。

## Useful Expressions

What type of gun was used?

使用的是什么类型的枪支?

Where exactly was the patient shot? Can you show me?

病人被射中的位置在哪里,能为我指一下吗?

I'm going to apply pressure here to try to slow the bleeding.

我要按压病人的伤口来减缓出血。

I need to cut away some of the patient's clothing to fully assess the wound.

我需要剪开病人的部分衣物来全面评估伤口。

The patient seems to lose a lot of blood.

病人看起来失血很多。

I'm concerned the bullet may have hit the patient's lung / liver / femoral artery, so we need to get him / her to the hospital quickly.

我担心子弹可能击中了病人的肺 / 肝 / 股动脉,所以我们需要尽快将他 / 她送往医院。

---

🔍 **Key Words and Phrases**

**femoral** [ˈfemərəl] adj. 股骨的,大腿骨的,大腿的;n. 股动脉

**artery** [ˈɑːtəri] n. 动脉

We're going to stabilize the patient's neck / back / limbs before transporting him / her to the hospital.

我们要固定住病人的颈椎 / 脊柱 / 肢体，然后才能把他 / 她送往医院。